Inducing Labour
Making Informed Decisions

This book replaces Induction: do I really need it?

Sara Wickham

Association for Improvements in the Maternity Services

©AIMS 2014

This book replaces Induction: do I really need it?

Published by AIMS
www.aims.org.uk

ISBN 978 1 874413 31 8

Printed in Great Britain by
TJ International
www.tjinternational.ltd.uk

Acknowledgments

I would like to thank all of the women whose stories and experiences have helped inform this book, and the women who work tirelessly for AIMS with the goal of improving maternity care for all.

Special thanks to Nadine Edwards, Virginia Hatton, Vicki Williams, Beverley Beech, Jean Robinson, Debbie Chippington Derrick, Emma Ashworth, Chloe Bayfield and Judith Payne, Tasha Cooper and not forgetting to re-mention Alice Charlwood and Pat Thomas whose work on the first edition helped set the foundation for this updated version.

Cover illustration by Vicki Williams ©AIMS 2014.

About AIMS

The Association for Improvements in the Maternity Services (AIMS) has been at the forefront of the childbirth movement since 1960, run entirely by unpaid volunteers. Our day-to-day work includes providing independent support and information about maternity choices and raising awareness of current research on childbirth and related issues. AIMS actively supports parents and healthcare professionals who recognise that, for the majority of women, birth is a normal rather than a medical event.

Contents

'Care for pregnant women differs fundamentally from most other medical endeavours. "Routine" care during pregnancy and birth interferes in the lives of healthy people, and in a process which has the potential to be an important life experience. It is difficult to imagine the extent to which our efforts might, for example, disturb the development of a confident, nurturing relationship between the mother and baby. The harmful effects we measure in randomised trials are limited to those we have predicted may occur. Sometimes after many years unexpected harmful effects surface only because they are relatively common, or striking in their presentation. Many unanticipated harmful effects probably never come to light.

'For these reasons, interventions in pregnancy and childbirth need to be subjected to special scrutiny. Our guiding principle is to advise no interference in the process of pregnancy and childbirth unless there is compelling evidence that the intervention has worthwhile benefits for the mother and/or her baby – only then is there a good chance that benefits will outweigh both known adverse effects and those which may not have been thought of.'

(Hofmeyr et al 2008, pxiii).

AIMS Foreword

AIMS intention is to support all women to have empowering births. This book is for all pregnant women with concerns or questions about inducing labour. It provides the most up-to-date evidence we have to help decide whether it is right for you or not. Most inductions for longer pregnancies are now taking place before 42 weeks. Therefore, most of these babies are not actually even post-term or 'overdue' by medical definitions.

We are frequently contacted by women who are told ultrasound results give irrefutable evidence regarding their 'due date', even when they know to the hour when the pregnancy began, or they know that in their family normal pregnancies last 43 weeks. We hope this book illustrates the much greater variation in human gestation than implied by current limited concepts of 'normality' and explains the limitations of technology in estimating the age of a pregnancy.

We know from talking to women who contact us that there are often complex emotional, social and medical reasons why women feel they would like the baby induced. If you decide induction is right for you, this book can prepare you for what to expect and what questions to ask your care providers. We are also aware that sometimes women are manipulated into agreeing to an induction by health practitioners against their better judgement. This book also provides information and support if you decide to continue your pregnancy.

There is no law that requires you to agree to an induction at any given stage in your pregnancy. It is the woman, and the woman alone, who has the legal and moral right to consent to any treatment or intervention. Induction is your decision. It is your baby, your body, your birth.

Readers may also like to note that not all research quoted as medical evidence or given to women as a reason for induction is as robust as it could be. Just because research has been published in a respectable journal does not mean the conclusions are right, and especially that they are right for your case. As we shall show, each piece of research has to be looked at in the context of other work on the subject.

Author's Foreword

Induction of labour is an increasingly common intervention. At some point during their pregnancy, many women find themselves needing to make a decision about this or about something relating to it, such as whether to let their midwife do a stretch and sweep (see page 11). In a very small number of cases, induction can be life-saving for women or babies, but lots of people (including women, families, researchers, midwives and doctors) are concerned that far too many inductions are happening and think that this is causing much more harm than good (Simpson and Thorman 2005, Lothian 2006, Keirse 2010, Berkowitz 2011, Glantz 2012).

The reasons for the current high rate of induction are complex and interlinked, but we think that part of the reason for this trend is related to the emphasis placed on risk. Modern western societies have become very focused on attempting to reduce risk and trying to ensure safety (Murphy-Lawless 1998, Edwards 2008). This often leads to the view that it is better to do something than not, although when I talk with women and couples about whether and how risk management is used in their own workplace, lots of people roll their eyes and almost everyone has a story about how this approach can lead to more problems than it solves in pretty much every field that you can think of.

Some people say the same about the risk management approach taken in maternity care.

Induction of labour is almost always carried out in an attempt to reduce risk. Sometimes this risk is an individual one, for instance where a woman who has been admitted to hospital with pre-eclampsia is told that it may be better if her labour is induced because the results of today's tests are more worrying than yesterday's. But most (if not all) areas also have standard guidelines which suggest that all women in particular groups should be offered induction of labour. The groups who are likely to be affected by these guidelines vary a bit according to which area you live in (Glantz 2012), but examples include women who have reached a certain week in their pregnancy, women who are deemed overweight or women who are older. The idea that a woman's labour should be induced if her pregnancy is 'prolonged' is so common that many women automatically assume that they will be induced on a certain date if they have not gone into labour on their own.

I did say that the reasons for induction of labour are complex, and it is important to mention that induction of labour (which allows people to predict roughly when women will give birth) may occasionally also be more convenient for the hospital, midwife or doctor. Sometimes women request induction themselves. Women can face a lot of pressure from all sorts of people towards the end of pregnancy ('haven't you had it yet?'). Perhaps this is because our modern culture values efficiency and productivity, because being overdue in any context is seen as a negative thing. But women have the right to make their own decision about this and any other issue, and the guidelines are just that: a guide. It can be just as reasonable to decide to wait for labour to start naturally, and in most cases most professionals will support women who make clear decisions that they do not want an intervention that is being offered. As I will explain in this book, the research evidence does not always support the viewpoint that it is better to intervene, and things are not always as clear-cut as some sources of information might suggest.

Before you read on, though, I would like to briefly introduce myself and to tell you a few things about me. This is because I believe it is important to be able to consider any information in the light of knowing who has written it and what their beliefs and perspective might be. Firstly, I am a midwife who believes that it is generally better not to intervene unless it is really warranted. I have also written lots of papers expressing the view that we induce labour far too often (Wickham 2007, 2009, 2010, 2011, 2012a, 2012b) and I wrote my PhD thesis on midwives' knowledge of post-term pregnancy.

My aim in writing this book, however, is not to persuade you to my way of thinking. I passionately believe that all women have the right to make the decisions that are right for them, their babies and families. I cannot possibly know what the best decision is for you, but I can try to guide you through some of the key information in this area. I can signpost other resources where they exist, and hopefully provide a woman-centred counterbalance to the people, information leaflets and websites that take the view that induction of labour is a wholly good thing which should be routine. This book has also been reviewed and edited by a whole committee of lovely people at AIMS who are committed to making sure that we have done our best to create something that will help you decide what course of action (or perhaps inaction) is best for you, your baby and your individual circumstances.

This book was first published in 2004, and AIMS and I sought lots of feedback before embarking on this updated edition. It became clear that, in several sections, we simply needed to update what was already there, while other parts of the book have undergone more extensive change and/or have been added or deleted because of changes in practice or the emergence of new research evidence. The format of the book has become simpler as a result, and it is now divided into three sections. The first gives an overview of the 'ins and outs' of induction, the second explores the decision process and the third looks at the research evidence in different areas. The book ends with the usual smorgasbord of references and resources to follow up if you are interested.

We know that it is really useful to be able to read women's own stories about their experiences, and the first edition of the book contained a few of these. We wanted to include more in this edition but had to consider its length. So, rather than make the book unwieldy or restrict the stories we included, we decided to create a related web page where you can read about other women's experiences of decision-making, waiting and induction, and/or share your own experience. We would encourage you to visit it at www.aims.org.uk.

My own website www.sarawickham.com also contains several relevant blog posts, a number of free articles and links to a lot of the documents mentioned in this book, and a page of updates can be found at www.aims.org.uk/pubsUpdates. You might also want to consider joining AIMS if you are not already a member, as this will mean you receive the AIMS Journals, which often contain updates and details of the latest research in this and other areas. It will also allow you to become a member of the AIMS discussion group.

Introduction

The dictionary definition of induce generally refers to bringing on, causing and bringing about, and the expression induction of labour is commonly understood to mean the bringing on of labour in a woman who was not previously showing any of the signs of labour, such as contractions.

Induction of labour is not the same as the acceleration (or augmentation) of labour, where a woman's labour is speeded up. This can be confusing, because augmentation of labour often uses the same drugs and techniques that are used to induce labour. But the key difference is that the word induction is used to describe the procedures used when labour hasn't already started on its own.

Rightly or wrongly, women, midwives and healers have used their knowledge of herbs, physical techniques and traditional therapies to bring on labour for thousands of years (Oteri and Tasker 1997, van der Kooy 1994). But, while the idea of trying to bring on labour might not be new, medical induction is a relatively recent phenomenon, and the reasons for inducing labour and the frequency with which this is done have changed dramatically over time.

In 2012-13, 23.3% of women who gave birth in England had their labour medically induced (NHS Maternity Statistics 2013). In Scotland the rate was 23.8% in 2011-12 (ISD Scotland 2013). This is more than one in five of all labours and births. The rate of induction and the reasons given for doing it seems to vary according to geographical area, and even between doctors working in the same hospital. For instance, the website www.birthchoiceuk.com shows that, in 2011, the Great Western Hospital in Swindon had the highest induction rate in England, at 37.2%, while Huddersfield Royal Infirmary had the lowest rate, at 5.2%.

This is important to bear in mind if someone suggests your labour should be induced. While one source of information might tell you that labour should be induced at 41 weeks if the baby hasn't been born, you may find that another sees no need for induction before 42 or more weeks of pregnancy unless there is a problem. Some women don't have their babies until they reach 43 or 44 weeks of pregnancy or later. There are no hard and fast facts here, and, even if there were, the decision is yours. As I will discuss later in this book, different people and places interpret the same research findings differently and take different approaches to the care they give. Some of the publications that I will discuss in this book seem to suggest that more inductions are better, yet American Professor of Obstetrics and Gynecology J Christopher Glantz (2012: 286-7) notes that, *'obstetrics has become ever more inclined toward increased intervention in recent decades'* despite the fact that *'no ascribable improvement has occurred in overall neonatal mortality, which has gradually declined since 1990 irrespective of whether the cesarean section rate rose or fell.'*

Most midwives and doctors are kind, caring people who want to support women and who respect their decisions. But it can sometimes be hard to always act in a caring way if you work in a system that is dominated by rules and in which you can get into trouble if you do not toe the line. Unfortunately, we know from experience that some doctors and midwives are more nervous than others about risk and they sometimes use scary and emotional language to express their concerns, telling women that induction is essential to save the life of their baby. Not to put too fine a point on it, some women have been told that their baby could die or that Social Services will be called if they do not consent to intervention.

This flies in the face of professional recommendations as well as your rights and if you have concerns about this then you can contact AIMS via one of the methods listed at the end of this book. But please understand that, while it is important to know what to do if this happens, this situation is occasional and the vast majority of healthcare professionals are reasonable and respectful of women's choices.

If you are offered induction, you should ensure that you ask as many questions as you need to. It is worth finding out what usually happens in your area and what the process would be in the hospital you might go to, and it is almost always possible to go home and take some time to discuss this with your partner or a relative or friend before making this important decision.

Part One

What Does Induction Involve?

Since childbirth became more medicalised, methods of inducing labour have become more sophisticated and invasive. This part of the book is designed to help you understand what induction involves and what questions you might want to ask if you are offered this. It begins with a quick introduction to natural labour, which provides a context for discussing each of the methods currently used in medical induction. Then there are sections on the location and timing of induction, induction and monitoring and the differences between spontaneous labour and induced labour. I haven't mentioned non-medical methods of inducing labour in this part, but will discuss those later on in the book.

A quick introduction to spontaneous labour

You may already know this bit, but I think it is useful to have a sense of what happens when a woman goes into labour spontaneously, because this can help us understand what needs to be done to induce labour artificially. Judith Lothian (2006: 43) suggested that:

'To make an informed decision—either informed consent or informed refusal—women need to know the value of waiting for labor to start on its own. The last days and weeks of pregnancy are vitally important for both the mother and her baby. The end of pregnancy is as miraculous as

5

its beginning. It's a lot easier to say "no" to induction if the mother knows the essential and amazing things that are happening to prepare her body and her baby for birth.'

(Judith's article is available free online at www.ncbi.nlm.nih.gov/pmc/articles/PMC1595289/ and it contains more information about this.)

During late pregnancy and early labour, loads of amazing things happen. Women pass antibodies to their baby, they might experience a nesting urge and they might also experience the insomnia that Judith Lothian (2006) suggests is the start of preparation for parenting (with which you may or may not agree!) While this is only one element of the whole, changes also happen in the woman's cervix, or neck of the womb. Firstly, it becomes softer and moves forward. This is the result of naturally occurring hormones and processes and is also influenced by the baby, although we actually know relatively little about the onset of natural labour and we most certainly can't predict when it will start in a particular woman. Cervical changes might happen at the same time as nesting for some women, while others will need longer. In the same way, natural labour begins slowly for some women, perhaps with the finding of a plug of bloody mucus when they visit the toilet and with the slow and gradual onset of cramping pains during the night, while for other women natural labour starts more suddenly, perhaps as their waters break with a gush.

No matter how labour starts, the process of natural labour causes further changes in the woman's cervix, which has already started to prepare for labour during the last few weeks of pregnancy. Her cervix moves forward, thins (effaces) and opens (dilates), so that the baby can begin to pass through the birth canal. The muscles of her uterus (womb) start to contract – perhaps irregularly at first, and then more regularly and strongly as labour progresses. These contractions cause her cervix to be drawn up and the baby to move down, and the baby's head (or sometimes the baby's bottom in the case of a breech) puts gentle pressure on her cervix, causing it to open further. This all happens in tandem with a cocktail of naturally-occurring hormones, including oxytocin, which helps facilitate all of these changes, and endorphins, which help relieve pain and create good feelings; some people describe these as nature's reward for being in natural labour!

Again, loads of other things happen in other dimensions, and I really don't want to suggest that the experience of labour and birth is all about the uterus. Nothing could be further from the truth, and in my view it is because labour and birth is such a holistic and complex whole-being experience that it can be so hard to induce medically, because this procedure focuses on only the physical aspects of this experience. But we have to consider the uterus – and initially the cervix – closely in this section, because it is the uterus that is the focus of medical induction. The key elements of natural labour that medical methods of inducing labour seek to replicate are the thinning, stretching and opening of the woman's cervix, hopefully alongside the bringing down of the baby's head, and the initiation and continuation of uterine contractions.

How is labour induced medically?

This section looks at the most commonly-used methods that are used to try to induce these elements of labour. I have divided these into three sections, because the first stage of induction – cervical ripening – can be achieved by more than one method. Different women who have their labours induced are likely to experience different methods, depending on where they live and on their individual circumstances. If you are offered induction of labour and think you might decide to have this, it is important to ask what your caregivers are proposing, talk through what options you have and ensure you have enough information and are happy with the choices you are making.

Cervical ripening

Towards the end of pregnancy, a woman's cervix moves forward and becomes softer, stretchier and thinner, in preparation for labour. We often say that the woman's cervix is becoming 'riper', as the changes are a bit like the change that occurs when fruit ripens. Where labour is induced, this ripening process needs to be encouraged by artificial means. In order to induce labour, the midwife or doctor also needs to break her waters (membrane rupture, which is discussed from page 22) and, usually, start an oxytocin drip to stimulate contractions (discussed from page 25). But her cervix needs to be a little bit open in order for the midwife or doctor to reach the membranes and break the waters, and unless her cervix is ripe then even an oxytocin drip isn't sure to work and induction is likely to fail. This is why cervical ripening is an important first step if medical induction is chosen.

One method of cervical ripening, a stretch and sweep, may be offered in the community (for example in a woman's home or at an antenatal clinic). In fact, it is becoming very common for midwives to offer women a stretch and sweep procedure in late pregnancy, in the hope that this will help her cervix to ripen, hasten labour and avoid a longer pregnancy. (It is sometimes said that this will prevent the need for induction, but I feel that the word 'need' is used inappropriately here, because it implies that every woman will need induction, yet some women will not need it because they will have gone into labour spontaneously, or wouldn't decide to be induced at that point anyway. There is more about so-called prolonged pregnancy in part three.) So I have included the stretch and sweep procedure in this section as well, because it is actually a method of induction which, like any other, has risks and benefits.

Most of the pharmaceutical methods of cervical ripening that are discussed here are used only when a woman decides to have a formal induction in a hospital. The drugs used to do this are sometimes described as cervical ripening agents. However, some hospitals have a policy of suggesting that women go home for a few hours after they have been given cervical ripening agents, as long as everything is OK.

Before we look at the different methods of cervical ripening, though, I want to explain the Bishop score. This is a scoring system that is used to rate how ripe a woman's cervix is, where 0 means that her cervix is not ripe (or ready for labour) at all and 10 means that it is very ripe. A ripe cervix will be soft and stretchy; it will have moved forward in the vagina and be beginning to open. A woman's cervix will be evaluated frequently during the process of induction, and the Bishop score will be one of the factors used to decide what the best next step is at any point.

Understanding the Bishop score

The Bishop score is worked out by assessing five elements of the state and position of your cervix and your baby during vaginal examination. Remembering how the cervix needs to get softer, stretchier and so on, the five things that are evaluated are:

The position of the cervix: before labour, the cervix tends to be further back (posterior) and it moves forward (anterior) as you go into labour.

The consistency of the cervix: this varies a bit depending on whether you have had a baby before, but cervixes become softer as labour nears and progresses.

The effacement of the cervix: again, this varies if you have had a baby before, but effacement describes the way in which the cervix becomes thinner and stretchier as labour nears and progresses.

The dilation of the cervix: the cervix opens (dilates) as labour progresses in order for the baby to move through it.

The fetal station: this describes how low in the pelvis the baby's head (or bottom in the case of a breech baby) is. As labour nears and progresses, the baby moves down and the lower down it can be felt, the higher the score that is given for this element.

Although there is some variation between different hospitals, a score of between 0 and 2 is given for each of these elements, with a higher score indicating that element is more favourable for labour. Generally, a score of above 8 is taken to indicate that the cervix is ripe and that induction has a good chance of working. Like any screening test, this is not perfect as a method of prediction (Verhoeven et al 2013). Women considering induction of labour many want to ask for information on the scoring system used locally and what this means in their particular case.

In some hospitals, doctors have started to consider using transvaginal ultrasound to evaluate the woman's cervix before and/or during induction of labour. However, a review by Verhoeven et al (2013) found no evidence that this is clinically useful in predicting the likely success of induction. It is also an unpleasant procedure and some women find it extremely distressing.

Stretch and sweep

It has now become common to offer women one or more stretch and sweeps in late pregnancy. During a vaginal examination, a midwife or doctor will sweep a finger around the opening of the woman's cervix in an attempt to stimulate contractions. A review of the research on this topic by Boulvain et al (2005) found that this is effective in bringing on labour a bit sooner than otherwise would be the case although eight women need to have a stretch and sweep in order to prevent one induction of labour. (Again, this figure assumes that all women would decide to have induction, which is not the case in reality.) Risks and downsides of a stretch and sweep are that it can cause discomfort, bleeding and irregular contractions, and in some of the studies the stretch and sweep intervention only brings labour forward by about 24 hours. The authors of this review concluded that:

'Routine use of sweeping of membranes from 38 weeks of pregnancy onwards does not seem to produce clinically important benefits. When used as a means for induction of labour, the reduction in the use of more formal methods of induction needs to be balanced against women's discomfort and other adverse effects.' (Boulvain et al 2005: 2)

Some midwives – with very good intentions – will offer a stretch and sweep procedure during an antenatal visit without much prior discussion, so it can be useful to have thought about whether you would want to have one or not ahead of time.

Prostaglandin

Labour can also be induced with the help of a number of pharmaceutical drugs, and the first of these that we will look at is prostaglandin, a drug that mimics the prostaglandin hormones produced naturally by the woman's body which causes her cervix to ripen and begin to open. Pharmacological versions of prostaglandins are used widely in labour induction, generally in the form of a pessary, tablet or gel, which is placed high in the vagina during vaginal examination, usually with the aid of plastic applicators (similar in size to a plastic tampon applicator).

Usually (though not always, according to women AIMS have talked to) before this or any of the next three methods are used, a vaginal examination is performed to assess the state of a woman's cervix. Consent should always be obtained before a vaginal examination is done. The midwife or doctor will feel the position, length, softness and openness of the cervix and, sometimes, each of these factors will be rated on a chart to form what is called a Bishop or cervical score, which was explained further on page 10. These scores are used to assess how ripe the woman's cervix is, and they can tell caregivers a few things about how successful induction is likely to be. In some areas the score may determine which method of induction is offered.

Prostaglandin gels, pessaries or tablets are inserted during a vaginal examination. The midwife or doctor will slide the applicator along their fingers until they can feel it is in the correct place, then release the pessary or gel and remove the applicator and their fingers. Some forms of prostaglandin work better if you remain lying down for a while after they are inserted so that they stay in the right place. Your midwife should tell you about this and ensure that you are comfortable (and that you have had a chance to go to the toilet) before this is inserted.

Because prostaglandins can cause strong contractions quickly, they can make it harder for the baby to cope, so monitoring will be recommended for around 30 minutes to an hour to check that the baby's heartbeat remains within normal limits (see page 37 for more on this). Once your caregiver has ensured that you and the baby are OK, it can then be a good idea to walk around for a bit and try to further stimulate contractions. However, women whose labours are induced may find they are advised to be continually monitored, and may not be able to move around as much as they need to, because of drips, fetal monitor belts and sometimes a variety of other equipment such as blood pressure machines. While it is always good to question whether such equipment or monitoring is necessary, it is important to remember that induction involves the use of strong drugs which can affect the woman and her baby.

Prostaglandins come in a variety of commercial brands; some examples include Prostin®, Dinoprostone® and Prepidil®. The amount and number of doses of prostaglandin that a woman is given will depend on whether she has had a baby before or if this is her first. It may also, as above, depend on how her cervix responds; for instance whether the Bishop score has changed. The process of assessing a woman's cervix and giving gels or pessaries may be repeated a few hours later, until her cervix is ripe enough for her waters to be broken.

Prostaglandins can cause pain in the form of a short period of intensely painful contractions, sometimes called 'prostin contractions'. While these contractions do not usually last for long, it can be tempting to think that contractions this painful must be dilating the cervix rapidly. This is not usually the case. Because having prostaglandins also involves having at least one vaginal examination, there is always a risk of introducing infection. Other side effects include:

- nausea and vomiting;

- diarrhoea;

- slight increase in temperature;

- hypotension (lowering of blood pressure);

- increased need for pain relief compared with when labour begins naturally;

- uterine hyperstimulation (where contractions become extremely strong);

- fetal distress;

- very rarely, uterine rupture – a serious condition necessitating emergency surgery;

- many women report that vaginal examination is more painful than usual following the administration of prostaglandins.

Some of the pharmaceutical companies issue cautions and a list of circumstances where they do not recommend the drug is used. For example:

- in women who have previously had a caesarean section or major uterine surgery;

- in women who are pregnant with more than one baby;

- in women who have polyhydramnios (an excess of amniotic fluid);

- in women whose membranes have already ruptured;

- in women whose baby's head has not yet engaged in their pelvis;

- in women who have had unexplained bleeding during pregnancy;

- in women who have epilepsy.

It is important to acknowledge, however, that any discrepancy between these recommendations and the way that prostaglandins (or any other drugs) are used in practice are not necessarily down to recklessness or ignorance on the part of the midwife, doctor or hospital. All of the drugs used in induction are associated with significant safety concerns but most of them have been used for years. While they are almost certainly overused, some of the exclusions are the result of caution on the part of pharmaceutical companies, who have not carried out appropriate research on the use of the drugs in pregnant women. The exception to this is misoprostol, which is associated with very significant safety concerns, as discussed next.

A note from AIMS for those with allergies, those who practise abstinence diets (for example, vegetarians), those with religious food practices and anyone who just wants to know what they are taking into their bodies.

Unlike laws for food labelling in the UK, there is no similar requirement for medicine.

Drug information sheets are included with all medicines and we recommend that you read them carefully before taking the drug and tell the doctor any information that may be relevant.

However, it is likely that you will only be shown this information sheet by hospital staff if you ask to see it.

Medicines are only required to give details of 'active ingredients' they contain, which must be listed on the drug information sheet. Medicines will also have 'inactive ingredients', which are components of the drug that generally do not increase or affect the therapeutic action of the active ingredient. Inactive ingredients are used to make the tablets or solutions that contain the drugs, and to make those that need to be swallowed palatable (such as coating of tablets). Examples include binding agents, dyes, preservatives and flavouring. It is possible that these inactive ingredients may cause allergic or adverse reactions.

It is extremely difficult to find out whether any medicines have active or inactive ingredients that are made from animal products or other ingredients that may be unacceptable to some people.

If you are told a drug is synthetic, it may still be animal derived. Chemical synthesis is often very complicated and using an animal source may make the production easier and hence cheaper, or there may be no suitable chemicals to use in the production process that can be obtained from plants. If a drug has been manufactured abroad, such as in China, details of the source may not be available.

The advice given to AIMS by a drugs company is to phone them direct to find out what was used to make each individual drug you wish to know about. You would need to do so for each different batch of drugs, because the ingredients could vary between batches of the same drug, although the quantity of the active ingredient would stay the same.

Please note that medical staff and midwives are unlikely to know whether the drug contains 'ingredients' that you wish to avoid or not. The information is not on the patient information sheet (there are no requirements for it to be) and neither is it in the British National Formulary (the book and website they use to obtain information about drug constituents – see www.bnf.org.) Ask for written information if staff claim knowledge.

It may be worth speaking to a pharmacist, either your local one or the hospital pharmacist, as they are likely to know more about the drug – although their sources of information are likely to be the same. Again, check their knowledge and ask for written information.

Be aware, also, that you may be obtaining information about a drug with a certain brand name, however, the NHS may prescribe you another cheaper version containing the same drug, but with different inactive ingredients. If so, you will have to start your checks all over again.

There are three useful websites where you may find information – an American one www.drugs.com and two UK ones www.medicines.org.uk and www.mhra.gov.uk/#page=DynamicListMedicines.

Misoprostol

In the last edition of this book, we discussed a drug called misoprostol, a less commonly used form of prostaglandin which can be administered via the vagina, in the rectum or by mouth. At that time, some doctors were advocating its widespread use for labour induction because it is cheaper and easier to administer and store than other prostaglandin drugs, but a number of people were campaigning for this to stop because of concerns about very serious side effects.

While it may still be used in medical delivery of the placenta, especially in low-income countries, where the risks appear to be less, many UK hospitals have stopped using misoprostol for induction. This is because of the very real danger that it can overstimulate the uterus, which in extreme cases has led to hysterectomy and maternal death. However, we cannot be certain that misoprostol is not still being used in some hospitals or in research studies.

The concerns about the use of misoprostol are so great that we would urge you to seriously question this if you are offered it. Because members of the AIMS committee know of cases where women have been given misoprostol without their knowledge or consent, however, we would advise any woman who decides to have her labour induced to ensure that she asks beforehand about what drugs will be used and makes it clear if there are any drugs that she would not wish to have.

More information on the dangers of misoprostol is discussed on websites such as www.inamay.com, www.midwiferytoday.com and www.sarawickham.com. Specific examples of articles can be found at www.midwiferytoday.com/articles/midwivescytotec.asp and www.midwiferytoday.com/articles/cytotec.asp. In the US, this drug is called cytotec, so if you are searching the internet on this subject I would recommend using both misoprostol and cytotec as search terms.

Foley catheters and laminaria tents

Over the past few years, the use of mechanical methods such as Foley catheters or laminaria tents to start labour has become more common. Although in the UK the current NICE guidelines recommend that these are not used routinely, they are in occasional use in some areas of the UK, in more frequent use in some other countries and gaining in popularity, so I felt the need to include information on them. These methods were popular many years ago (and in fact are variations of the first induction methods used) but they fell out of fashion because they were a common source of infection. Modern sterilisation methods mean that the infection risk is reduced and it is now possible that they may become more popular again. Both of the methods described in this section are physical devices which sit in or above the woman's cervix and are designed to stretch it open.

Foley catheters are the kind of catheters that are also used in people's bladders. A Foley catheter consists of a silicone or rubber tube which has a small balloon on the end that sits inside the body. Once the tube is in place, the balloon is inflated by filling it with a sterile saline solution to stop it from slipping out. In induction of labour, the end of the catheter is inserted through the neck of the womb and the midwife or doctor will then fill the balloon with saline from the other end of the catheter using a syringe. The idea is that the inflated balloon will perform a similar action to the baby's head and put pressure on the woman's cervix from the inside, thus encouraging it to open. Sometimes, the end of the catheter will be taped to the woman's leg to put a bit of pressure on her cervix. In some areas, practitioners advocate adding weights to the catheter or pulling on it every so often in order to further encourage the cervix to open. We do not yet have enough research to know whether Foley catheters are effective, although the results of some recent small studies are not promising, in that women seem to be in labour for longer than if they had had prostaglandin (Jozwiak et al 2011, Henry et al 2013). Mechanical methods of induction may, however, be an alternative for women who do not want to have prostaglandins.

Laminaria tents (also described as rods, cones or sticks) are thin sticks of a kind of dried seaweed which expands when it comes into contact with fluid, such as that secreted in the vagina. One or more can be inserted into the woman's cervix and they will then expand over several hours and, again, cause the cervix to dilate. They have a thread attached to one end, like a tampon, and a collar at the other end which is designed to prevent them entering the womb itself.

The main side effects of both Foley catheters and laminaria tents are infection and pain. Even though better sterilisation methods are now available for the devices themselves, anything that is put into the vagina (including gloved fingers and the jelly and/or fluid used during vaginal examination) has the potential to alter the balance of the normal bacteria in the vagina or to introduce different bacteria, both of which can cause infection. In some women, the latex found in some gloves and catheters can also cause irritation and/or inflammation. The results of a review of research into mechanical methods of induction of labour by Jozwiak et al (2012) found that the chances of having a caesarean section were pretty much the same for women who had mechanical methods and women who had prostaglandin. A study from Japan showed that overinflating the balloon catheter led to a greater risk of cord prolapse, which in turn led to a higher risk of cerebral palsy in the baby (Yamada et al 2013). Cord prolapse can also be caused by artificial rupture of the membranes. Mechanical methods appeared to be better than prostaglandins in that there were fewer cases of women having excessive uterine contractions. More research needs to be done to look at the rate of infection and also at the degree of pain women experience. It is important to remember, as above, that prostaglandins can also be painful. It is almost impossible to know from research which of these methods is more painful, and it is likely that this will vary between individual women.

Membrane rupture

Sometimes, a woman's waters (or membranes) break (or rupture) during the process of cervical ripening. But more often, once the Bishop score indicates that the woman's cervix is ripe enough for labour, then the next step in the induction process will be to break her waters artificially. This procedure may be described as artificial rupture of membranes, ARM, breaking the waters or amniotomy. It is almost always performed during a vaginal examination (unless the bag of membranes is so low that it is protruding from the vagina, which is extremely unlikely in the majority of cases of induction) and it can only be carried out if the woman's cervix is open and/or stretchy enough to allow the practitioner to reach the bag of waters and touch it with their fingers. For some women, especially those having their second or subsequent baby, their cervix will be ripe enough that their waters can be broken without using prostaglandins or mechanical methods first, but it is more common, especially in women having their first baby, to need to have cervical ripening methods first.

Because breaking the waters can sometimes cause distress to the baby, the baby's heartbeat should be checked before and after the procedure, although AIMS is aware that this does not always happen in practice.

With two fingers inside the vagina, the midwife or doctor will slide a long, flat plastic amnihook (like a long flattened crochet hook) along their fingers to reach the bag of waters. The top of the hook is rounded so that it does not hurt the woman, but just underneath this top part is a small sharp edge. Once it is in place against the bag of waters, the hook is then turned so that the sharp part pierces the membranes. As a midwife, I can tell you from experience that this sometimes takes several attempts, so the vaginal examination may last for longer than normal. In some areas, a thimble-like tool called an amnicot will be used on the midwife or doctor's finger to break the bag of waters, again during a vaginal examination. Whenever the bag of waters is broken, the midwife or doctor should keep their fingers inside the vagina for a few seconds to check that the baby's head comes down safely and that the cord does not move in front of the head, causing a cord prolapse. When this happens, the cord falls down below the baby's head and this means that the baby's head cannot pass through the woman's pelvis without squashing the cord. This would restrict the blood flow in the cord, causing the baby to receive a reduced supply of oxygen. A cord prolapse usually results in an emergency caesarean section. Women should be aware that the need to check that the cord has not prolapsed also means that the vaginal examination might last longer than is usual.

For a few women, having their waters broken (with or without having had prostaglandins or mechanical ripening methods first) may be enough to start labour, and practitioners will usually wait at least a couple of hours to see if this happens. For many women, however, labour will not become well-enough established within the time given, and an intravenous oxytocin drip is the next step in the process of induction.

Like other methods of labour induction, artificial rupture of membranes (ARM) can:

- speed up contractions;

- cause pain to increase faster than if you were in spontaneous labour;

- increase the risk of infection and umbilical cord prolapse (where the cord slips in front of the baby's head necessitating an immediate emergency caesarean) – though this is rare;

- cause fetal distress.

Once ARM has been performed, caregivers will tend to take the position that everyone is now committed to the continuation of the induction, since the risk of infection to the baby is increased by breaking the waters. This, then, also carries the chance that, if the ARM and concurrent methods of inducing labour are not successful, the woman may be offered a caesarean section. However, it is important to remember that all of this is the woman's decision and it is important to ask why it is being offered, what the risks are and whether the situation is an emergency or if it is possible to wait a few hours to think about things, to see if labour continues on its own and/or to try again after having a rest.

Stimulating contractions

In natural labour, the hormone oxytocin − also known as the hormone of love! − is secreted by the pituitary gland. Oxytocin is responsible for the creation and continuance of the contractions of the muscles in the uterus which further open the woman's cervix and allow the baby to move through the birth canal. See the box on page 26 for a little more about natural oxytocin. A synthetic form of this hormone has also been created and this drug is used to stimulate contractions in women having their labour induced. This oxytocin needs to be given into a vein so that it goes directly into the woman's bloodstream and so it is given via an intravenous or IV drip. There couldn't be more contrast, however, between the way in which natural oxytocin is coming to be seen as a marvellous hormone which plays an enormous part in our relationships (Uvnäs-Moberg 2003, 2011) and the way in which Korte and Scaer (1984) quote Roberto Caldeyro-Barcia, a former president of the International Federation of Gynecology and Obstetrics (FIGO), as having said that synthetic oxytocin is *the most abused drug in the world today.'*

Oxytocin: the hormone of love

Oxytocin in its natural form is often described as the hormone of love, hugs, bonding and/or cuddles. We have known for a while that it plays an important part in sex, birth, breastfeeding and bonding, and more recent research shows that it is also involved in orgasm, friendship, social relationships and in helping us cope with stress. It can reduce fear, hostility and depression, it relieves pain and it plays a role in weight loss.

Natural oxytocin can be generated by actions as simple as shaking hands or hugging, and many research studies are being carried out to explore the already vast array of human behaviours and situations in which this hormone is involved. It is almost certain that we will keep learning much more about this over the next few years.

It is important to know that, unfortunately, while synthetic oxytocin clearly has some uses in medicine, it inhibits our body's ability to release natural oxytocin. (This is one reason why it is really not advisable to try and birth your placenta naturally if you have had oxytocin to induce or augment your labour). There are also concerns about the effect that synthetic oxytocin has on the number of oxytocin receptors that we have in our bodies, and whether having synthetic oxytocin during one labour may have an impact on your future labours too. Some people are very concerned about our overuse of synthetic oxytocin during labour and birth and if you would like to find out more then is it worth checking out the work of Uvnas-Moberg (2011), Michel Odent (2009, 2010a, 2010b) and Buckley (2009), whose books and articles are all listed in the reference list. Some of Sarah Buckley's work can also be found at www.sarahbuckley.com.

The artificial form of oxytocin is also known as syntocinon in the UK and pitocin in the US and is often abbreviated by midwives and doctors to synto, synt and/or pit. Synthetic oxytocin is given to try to induce or speed up labour, but it is important to know from the outset that this does not always work. Some people think that this is because the baby or the woman is not yet ready for labour. This is discussed further below. Conversely, if synthetic oxytocin does produce contractions, they can become much stronger and more painful more quickly than the contractions of spontaneous natural labour. Some women request that the speed of the drip be turned down if the contractions become too overwhelming.

If a woman decides to have oxytocin, a needle will be used to insert a plastic cannula (fine tube) into her arm or hand and a bag of intravenous fluid containing the syntocinon will be attached to this, usually held on a pole. In order to control the strength and duration of syntocinon-induced contractions as much as possible (so as to keep the pain within a tolerable limit and because strong contractions can be hazardous to both mother and baby), the drip will be started at a slow rate and then gradually increased over time. As there are risks to using syntocinon, the woman's contractions and the baby's heartbeat will usually be monitored continuously once a drip has been started. The midwife should stop increasing the drip once a vaginal examination confirms that the contractions have become strong enough to be dilating the woman's cervix.

The risks of syntocinon are similar to the risks of prostaglandins, and include:

- headache;

- nausea and vomiting;

- arrhythmia, or irregular heartbeat;

- lowered blood pressure;

- bleeding;

- skin rashes;

- hyperstimulation of the uterus, causing very painful contractions which can cause the baby to become distressed;

- reduction in oxygen supply to the baby;

- uterine rupture;

- increased risk of blood clots after birth;

- increased risk of urinary incontinence in later life;

- interference with the body's ability to produce its own oxytocin, which is why a managed birth of the placenta is recommended.

Vaginal examinations (VEs) are usually performed fairly frequently throughout the entire induction process, but perhaps even more so while synthetic oxytocin is being given so that the midwife can find out if the woman's cervix is dilating in response to the drug. (See the box below for more information about vaginal examination.) The baby's heartbeat will also be monitored continuously after the drip is started to keep an eye on whether the baby becomes distressed. If the woman decides to have pain relief, this may involve other kinds of monitoring; for instance, women who have epidurals need to have their blood pressure monitored regularly because the drugs given by the epidural route can have an effect on their blood pressure.

Vaginal examination

A woman whose labour is being induced will often have many vaginal examinations during the process. Staff will want to examine her to find out whether her cervix is ripe, to do a stretch and sweep, and before they insert a gel, pessary or tablet, insert a mechanical cervical ripening device, break her waters or put up a drip. The actual insertion of a gel, pessary, tablet and/or mechanical cervical ripening device and the breaking of a woman's waters are both done via vaginal examination, as is the assessment of whether these have worked. If an oxytocin drip is put up, regular vaginal examination will be strongly recommended, sometimes every two hours, to assess progress. Vaginal examinations may also be advised if a woman requests pain relief or if there is concern about the baby's well-being.

Vaginal examinations can be embarrassing, uncomfortable, painful and/or distressing and they carry risks of introducing infection into the woman's vagina or uterus. They can have a negative psychological effect on women and this may impact on a woman's ability to labour effectively. Women have every right to ask if each vaginal examination is really necessary and can expect an explanation of why each vaginal examination is being recommended, and/or to ask that these be kept to a minimum. However, in our experience, this does not always happen. Women also have a right to refuse to have them although it is important to understand that some of the procedures listed above cannot be carried out other than during a vaginal examination. So it is not possible, for instance, to decline vaginal examination and still have your membranes ruptured. Women also have the right to ask for vaginal examinations to be carried out in positions other than on their back on the bed, especially if this position is uncomfortable. Some practitioners may say that this is too difficult for them to do – for instance if a woman is on all fours then what they are feeling is reversed, which may be difficult for inexperienced or less flexible practitioners. If this is the case, a good position to suggest is where the woman squats or kneels upright on the bed, perhaps supported by one or two companions, because the woman's vagina is then in almost the same place and position as if the woman was lying on the bed.

Women do not have to allow midwifery or medical students to examine them if they do not wish to. Although vaginal examinations are an integral part of the induction process, as they enable the administration of drugs and procedures and the assessment of progress, women have every right to decline or to negotiate with caregivers how often these are carried out, and by whom.

If the induction is successful, and labour progresses well, the baby can be born as usual. After the baby is born, it is highly likely that the midwife or doctor will want actively to manage the birth of the placenta (also called the third stage of labour). This involves keeping the syntocinon drip going, holding the uterus in place with one hand and pulling on the cord with the other to remove the placenta. While this is not the same as a physiological third stage (where the placenta is born naturally without the use of drugs or other midwife interventions), synthetic oxytocin inhibits the woman's body from releasing her own oxytocin and there is a significant chance that stopping or removing the oxytocin drip suddenly could lead to excessive bleeding.

Sometimes, women ask me whether they can have a physiological (natural) birth of the placenta after induction. Technically, you could ask for the synthetic oxytocin drip to be removed at any time, but it is advisable to reduce it slowly over a period of time because syntocinon disrupts the body's natural release of oxytocin and women who have had their labour induced or augmented are more likely to bleed heavily after birth. If you attempted to stop the drip suddenly in order to attempt a 'physiological' or natural birth of the placenta (although I really do not think it could reasonably be called that, as the labour itself wasn't physiological), there would be a likelihood of excessive bleeding. I have discussed this further at sarawickham.com/2013/11/11/can-i-have-a-natural-placental-birth-after-induction/.

I am sorry if the following statement sounds harsh, but I think it is important to recognise that induction of labour is a serious intervention which is best thought of as a 'package deal'. Although there are some choices to be made along the way, some of the core elements of it (including repeated vaginal examinations, ongoing monitoring and management of elements of labour, such as the birth of the placenta) are an intrinsic and inseparable part of that package. It is important that women who are considering induction of labour understand this, as my experience tells me that this is not always explained well. In natural labour, it is possible and reasonable to question or decline any of the things mentioned above, and there is far more potential for making choices. This doesn't mean that you have no options if you decide to have an induction, but it is important to understand that it does make certain interventions advisable and/or intrinsically necessary.

If, however, labour became established after the use of cervical ripening and/or artificial rupture of membranes and no synthetic oxytocin was used, the situation around placental birth may be different, although I do not know of any research that has looked at this question either. Nadine Edwards and I (2011) wrote a book for AIMS about the third stage of labour, *Birthing Your Placenta – The Third Stage*, which provides more information on the birth of the placenta.

Even after the placenta has been delivered, because of the way in which synthetic oxytocin inhibits the woman's own production of this hormone, the drip is usually left on for up to an hour or more after the baby is born. The midwife will check that the woman's uterus is well contracted before the drip is finally stopped and taken out.

Failed induction

For some women, no amount of drugs will bring on labour, and the decision may be made that, despite all efforts, the induction has 'failed' and a caesarean section may be recommended. For others, the side effects of the drugs used may cause fetal distress or hyperstimulation of the uterus. Both of these are potentially serious situations likely to necessitate a caesarean delivery.

If the labour is not going well, if synthetic oxytocin can't generate strong enough contractions, if the baby or woman becomes distressed by the drugs or too tired by the length of the labour, it is likely that the midwife or doctor will suggest an instrumental or operative delivery, where a vacuum extractor or forceps or a caesarean section will be used to deliver the baby. If the woman's cervix has fully dilated by this point and the baby is in a good position and not too distressed, it may be possible to use instruments such as forceps or ventouse to deliver the baby. If the cervix has not fully dilated or if the baby is not in such a good position then a caesarean section may be the only option. Sometimes, one or more of these scenarios is called a failed induction, but it is important to remember that it is the system that has failed and not the woman. It also does not mean that she would have failed to go into labour or to labour effectively if the labour had been spontaneous.

If this happens — or has previously happened — to you, please do not think you have failed if your body does not go into labour, if your labour does not progress as fast as the professionals would like, or if your baby becomes distressed as a result of the drugs you have been given. Although the language used can sometimes make it sound as if it is your 'fault', it is western medicine and inductions which sometimes fail; women's bodies do not.

Where does induction take place?

As stated above, although a stretch and sweep is sometimes carried out in a community setting or at a woman's home, medical inductions almost always take place in hospital. Some hospitals have special areas where they administer prostaglandins and insert mechanical means of cervical ripening, but in others this happens on the antenatal ward. In a few places, some women can go home after a cervical ripening procedure. They will have an appointment to return a few hours later for assessment and further procedures, although of course they can return sooner if they go into labour or are worried. In others places women will be admitted to the antenatal ward straight away and will then stay in hospital until they have given birth.

Normally, women only go to the labour ward once labour has established, if pain relief becomes necessary or because more invasive procedures such as artificial rupture of membranes or intravenous oxytocin are indicated. (It is important to know, however, that women are sometimes refused certain kinds of pain relief until labour has become established.) In the vast majority of cases these procedures will be carried out on a labour ward because they have the potential to distress the baby and it is important to be near an operating theatre in case an emergency caesarean section becomes necessary. Women who have obstetric or medical complications may go straight to the labour ward when they come into the hospital. Some hospitals also have special areas close to the labour ward that are used just for women who are being induced.

Sometimes, women being induced are in a room with other women whose labours are also being induced. Women can request a private room, but one may not be available, or they may be told they need to pay for this. Privacy has been shown to be hugely important to labouring women, and labour often doesn't start (or if it has started, it may stop) in situations where women feel they are being observed.

A major problem for many women is that their partners or birth companions are not always allowed onto the antenatal ward or induction bay, or they might only be allowed to visit at certain times. Even if they are allowed there for some of the time, they usually have to leave overnight (which is often when women want them the most, especially if they are in pain). Partners can usually stay once a woman is on the labour ward, but women can be in early labour on the antenatal ward or in another area of the hospital for quite a while before this happens.

If you are offered induction, you may want to ask more about where you would be and for how long before you decide whether you would want this. Being unexpectedly separated can be distressing if you wanted your partner with you, and this can affect the progress of your labour, so you may want to discuss this with the hospital staff ahead of time. It may also be worth asking about the 'worst-case scenario' in terms of the timing – for example, what happens if it takes a couple of days for you to go into established labour – because some women do not realise that they might be separated from their partner and family for quite some time. Some women have had success in arguing the case for their partner to stay, especially if they make it clear that they do not want their labour to be induced unless this is made possible.

Does the time of day or night matter?

In most cases, the timing of induction is primarily determined by the policies and protocols of the hospital where the induction will take place. These are considered necessary because of the sheer numbers of women who give birth in each institution, and because of the need to manage the number of women and babies who are in different areas of the hospital (for example, the antenatal ward and the delivery suite) at any given time. However, it may be possible to negotiate on an individual basis.

A couple of reviews have looked at whether it makes a difference if induction of labour is started in the morning or the evening. Bakker et al (2013) analysed three research studies which compared women who had induction of labour beginning with prostaglandin. Some of the women were first given this in the morning and some had their first dose in the evening. The review found that the outcomes (in relation to safety) were the same no matter when the first dose of prostaglandin was given, but, in one of these studies, a significant number of the women who were given the first dose of prostaglandin in the evening reported dissatisfaction compared with the women who were given the first dose in the morning.

We can't be sure of exactly why this is, but I can speculate from my experience as a midwife. Evening induction was once thought to be good because the first dose of prostaglandin – which often takes time to work – would work overnight while the woman slept. But anyone who has tried to sleep in a hospital ward (and/or who has experienced the pain of prostaglandin-induced contractions) will know that the theory doesn't quite match the reality here. If a woman has made the decision to have her labour induced, she is likely to want to get on with it in the morning rather than waiting all day for it to begin, especially if she knows that she may not be sleeping much for the next few days. As a result of this and previous reviews, NICE (2008) guidelines recommend carrying out induction of labour with prostaglandin in the morning.

Induction and monitoring

Once the induction process has started, health professionals will want to monitor the progress of labour and the well-being of both the woman and her baby. As discussed in 'Understanding the Bishop score' on page 10, the main means of monitoring the progress of labour is to carry out regular vaginal examinations to assess the state of the woman's cervix and the position of the baby. The midwife or doctor will also ask about women's experience of contractions, they may ask to feel them with their hand and/or they can see how strong they are by using an electronic fetal monitor. (It is important to note, however, that electronic fetal monitors are not a very accurate way of measuring contractions.)

All hospitals are equipped with these cardiotocograph (CTG) monitors, which also measure the baby's heartbeat using ultrasound. Some hospitals use more complex monitoring systems, so you might want to ask what is used locally. Usually, the CTG transducers (the circular discs that transmit the ultrasound and pick up the heartbeat and contractions) are attached to the woman's abdomen with belts and left on, either for a while (intermittent monitoring) or continuously. Sometimes, the midwife or doctor will ask if they can monitor the baby's heartbeat using an internal monitor that is screwed into the baby's scalp. Intermittent monitoring can also be done using a Pinard (ear trumpet), a hand-held 'sonicaid' (another ultrasound device), or by the midwife holding one of the transducers from the CTG on your abdomen for a minute (rather than having it strapped to your abdomen with a belt).

The reason for monitoring is that all methods used in medical induction can cause the baby to become distressed. As mentioned previously, occasionally this distress can be sudden and lead to the need for an emergency caesarean section, so it is considered important to listen to the baby's heartbeat before, during and/or after each procedure.

The NICE guidance (2008, 2013) did not find any evidence relating to the effectiveness of different monitoring methods when labour is induced, and there is some variation in this between different hospitals. But it is fairly common practice that, when drugs such as prostaglandin are given, the baby's heartbeat and the woman's contractions will be monitored for at least 20–30 minutes before and after the procedure.

If labour becomes established without the use of synthetic oxytocin then intermittent monitoring may be offered, although if a woman has a synthetic oxytocin drip, continuous monitoring is likely to be recommended. As this involves the attachment of at least one transducer to the mother's abdomen by belts, and wires connecting the transducers and the CTG machine itself, it can be very difficult for the woman to walk around or to change position. This can be a cause of serious additional discomfort and sometimes distress to the woman, because moving around and changing position can reduce the pain of contractions. As a consequence of this, and the increased pain of contractions caused by artificial syntocinon, women are more likely to want an epidural – indeed, many hospitals will offer this at the same time as putting a syntocinon drip up.

Fetal monitoring is not an exact science. Occasionally there will be a 'false negative' trace where the baby will appear to be healthy on the monitor, but may actually be poorly when it is born. A far more common problem is with 'false positive' CTG traces, where the baby is thought to be distressed but is not. Sometimes this is thought to be a serious emergency and the woman is rushed into theatre for a caesarean section, yet the baby is delivered in perfectly good health.

While both AIMS and myself encourage women to question the need for intervention and monitoring in normal labour if it doesn't feel right for them, the situation is a little different when women are being induced. No woman should ever feel like she has to do something, but at the same time it is important to understand that medical induction poses significant risks to the baby and that, because of this, monitoring (like managed third stage) may be genuinely warranted where women decide to have induction of labour.

Comparing spontaneous labour and induced labour

All labours are different, so I should confess at the outset that I can't really offer the information that the title of this section implies, because each woman's experience is so individual, but according to women who have experienced both, there are some key differences between spontaneous and induced labour.

Spontaneous labour is less painful than induced labour. This may be partly because a labour that starts spontaneously usually builds up gradually, giving the woman time to get used to each new sensation, and is accompanied by the release of endorphins, which are natural substances that help relieve pain, but also because the amount of monitoring used in induced labour means that a woman's movement may be restricted.

This means that women whose labours are induced may be more likely to need pain relief than women who go into spontaneous labour, and will tend to use it at an earlier stage than women who are in spontaneous labour. Sometimes women whose labours are induced experience so much pain or discomfort during the process of cervical ripening that they ask to have an epidural sited at the same time as the syntocinon drip, because they cannot face the thought of more pain.

While it is great that modern medicine can provide such good methods of pain relief when it is needed, it is important to remember that all drugs have side effects. Sometimes the drugs used for the induction itself or for pain relief can have adverse effects on the woman or baby, and may lead to the need for further intervention.

Women who go into spontaneous labour and who are planning to give birth in hospital still usually spend at least some time at home or in their own environment and go to hospital when they are ready. This means that women who go into spontaneous labour tend to find the early part of this labour easier than women whose labour is induced, because instead of sitting in a hospital bed wondering how long it is going to take, they are still involved in normal life, which can make the first part of their labour pass more quickly and pleasantly.

Some women also experience psychological trauma and unwanted side effects after induction of labour. This can occur when labour starts spontaneously as well, but the increased interventions that are a part of induction may make this more likely when labour is induced. Some women find that the synthetic oxytocin, the tiredness caused by a long labour and/or the other drugs and interventions they experience lead them to have difficulties in bonding with the baby or establishing breastfeeding. Some women also feel that they were not in control of their birth experience, and this can sometimes lead to postnatal depression or even post-traumatic stress disorder.

Part Two

Making Decisions About Induction

In the UK, national guidelines place strong emphasis on the fact that midwives and doctors should help women to make informed decisions about their care or treatment, and suggest that *'healthcare professionals should explain the following points to women being offered induction of labour:*

- *the reasons for induction being offered;*

- *when, where and how induction could be carried out;*

- *the arrangements for support and pain relief (recognising that women are likely to find induced labour more painful than spontaneous labour);*

- *the alternative options if the woman chooses not to have induction of labour;*

- *the risks and benefits of induction of labour in specific circumstances and the proposed induction methods;*

- *that induction may not be successful and what the woman's options would be.'* (NICE 2008)

This part of the book goes into most of the main reasons that women are given as justification for an induction. This doesn't mean that they are all good reasons for induction – although some of them certainly can be for some mothers and babies. The aim of this part is to provide a reference guide for you to be able to find out more about any reasons you might be given for needing an induction, and information which might give you an idea of whether – or when – induction might be appropriate in your case. It also aims to help you ask relevant questions. Of course, it is impossible to write a book that can speak to every individual woman and take into account all the possible variations, so this is mainly intended as a starting point. You may also want to read some of the references and resources referred to in this book to find more information.

One thing to remember is that, if you are told your labour needs to be induced, it is hardly ever a dire emergency. If a doctor was worried that you or your baby were in any imminent danger, she would not be recommending induction of labour. She would be advising an immediate caesarean section. I think it is important to know this because some women attend an antenatal appointment or go to hospital to have the baby's heartbeat monitored and are told they need to stay and have their labour induced right away. Although there are a few exceptional cases where a woman or baby has a condition which is not immediately life-threatening but may become more dangerous over the next day or two (in which case immediate induction may be warranted), it is almost always possible to take some time to go home and think about the situation, gather more information and discuss it with your family or friends before you make a decision.

If caregivers are reluctant for you to go home for some reason, you could call someone to come and join you and go for a cup of tea in the cafeteria or a walk in the hospital grounds with them. You are also entitled to ask for a second opinion, and it might be helpful to ask to speak to a Supervisor of Midwives, a consultant midwife (if the unit has one) or a midwifery manager. There is more information on how to contact a Supervisor of Midwives on page 52.

Hospitals are bureaucratic institutions and, while it may be easier for the hospital to admit you immediately, you may want to think about other options, sort out your other commitments or simply take a little time to 'get your head around' what is being proposed and whether it is the best decision for you. The fact that women are sometimes given the impression that their labour needs to be induced immediately when this is not the case is well illustrated by Claire's story:

'I went to my antenatal and they said I should be induced … I already sort of knew that because they said it the last time as well when I saw the hospital. They said, "do you want to just stay in today 'cause we can fit you in?", so I thought I might as well, seeing as the kids were with my mum anyway.

'They were going to give me the gel that evening, but then they said they couldn't … I think that first time it was because there weren't enough midwives and too many women in labour already. So I thought, OK, well at least I'll get a good night's sleep. But of course you never do in hospital, do you?

'And this went on for two more days. They said the labour ward was full, and there were other women who were being induced as well. They wouldn't start us all off at the same time. Finally, when they gave me the gel, it was the Wednesday evening, and I'd gone in on the Monday morning. And I thought, well I might as well have been at home, left the kids with Mum and had a rest rather than sitting there. I know they're really busy, and the midwives did keep saying they were sorry, but it was always like, I couldn't go home because they thought they might start me off in the next few hours. I was a bit afraid if I did go home I might miss my place in the queue!

'That's the bit that I wish had been different. Because when I had the baby I was so tired from not sleeping that I'm sure I would have enjoyed the first few days more if that hadn't happened and I'd just come in when they were ready.'

Questions you may want to ask

As scientific studies show that too many inductions are happening routinely with no benefit to the mother or baby, if induction of labour is being suggested, there are some useful questions you could ask:

Why do you feel I need to be induced?

If you are clear on the specific reason (or reasons) for which induction is being recommended in your case, you can ask your caregivers to give you the evidence that supports their advice so that you can look at it and then make a more informed decision about what you would like to do.

Am I or my baby in imminent danger?

If this is the case then you may want to consider immediate induction. If not then you may want to take time to think about your options and talk to your family before you make a decision. If you are being told that you are putting your baby at serious risk and you suspect that this is being said to persuade you to agree to an induction, you can state that you want a second opinion. Some people believe that, if urgent delivery is indicated, it may even be better to consider a caesarean section.

What are the benefits of being induced for my specific situation?

This links with the first question above, and will give you a clearer picture about whether there is a specific reason why induction may be a good idea for you, or whether this is a routine recommendation. Being told 'Oh, it is something we always do for everyone who goes overdue' is not necessarily a good reason for inducing your baby.

What are the risks of being induced?

All medical procedures carry risks, and the specific risks of induction are discussed elsewhere in this book. Asking this question can help you determine whether a health professional is being honest with you, or whether they simply want you to do what they suggest, perhaps by toning down or denying that there are risks involved. If you are told that there are no real risks, you are being misled and you may want to seek a second opinion. If the professional concerned is a doctor, you may wish to talk to your midwife about your options; if it is a midwife, then you can ask to speak to the Supervisor of Midwives, see page 52 for information on how to contact your local SOM. You can also contact AIMS to talk things through.

What percentage of women who are induced in this hospital end up having a caesarean section or an instrumental birth (forceps or vacuum extraction)?

These figures should be available, and you should ask for the local statistics. You can also look at www.birthchoiceuk.com to see what the intervention (including induction) rates are for your local hospital, alongside national rates, which will give you an idea of the general philosophy and the likelihood of intervention in that unit generally. An operative or instrumental delivery is a very real risk of induction, and a professional who is being honest with you should acknowledge this, rather than glossing over the fact.

What kind of monitoring do you suggest for induction?

Most hospitals want to put continuous monitors on women who are having a syntocinon drip, and for a while after the administration of a gel (see page 13). You have the right to decline any monitoring or other interventions that the hospital offers although, as discussed on page 38, you should bear in mind that powerful drugs are used to induce labour and that these can sometimes cause harm or stress to babies. If you feel a health professional is not appropriately acknowledging the risks of induction, you can ask why they feel monitoring is so important, which will hopefully lead to a more honest discussion about the risks and benefits. A related important question is:

How do you adapt monitoring and other elements of the process to let women move around if they want to do this to help labour progress?

The best answer to this question will concern an honest discussion of positioning, monitoring and movement options that acknowledges the increased difficulty that occurs when women are being induced but gives realistic suggestions. Sadly, some units and professionals will tell women what they think they want to hear, so be wary of people who airily tell you that you can do anything you want or that it will be just as easy as if you were in spontaneous labour. It won't. You will need to negotiate the monitoring leads and, even if you spend most of the time standing up, you will get weary of being made to get on the bed every time someone wants to examine you or reposition the monitor, and some women eventually lose the energy to keep getting back off again.

What choices do I have if I choose to be induced?

If you think that induction may be genuinely warranted in your case, you may want to ask whether you have a choice in method of cervical ripening. This may lead to important differences, for instance in whether you can visit a cervical ripening clinic and then go home to await events, or whether one course of action is more likely to mean your partner can stay with you throughout.

What are the alternatives to being induced?

There may be an alternative to induction, depending on the reason(s) why it is being suggested. If there is concern about your or the baby's well-being, it may be possible to arrange regular monitoring instead, and to see how things go. Or you may want to consider a planned caesarean section instead. While you will want to take into account your caregiver's knowledge in this area, you will be able to tell from their response to this question how open they are to helping you explore the different options available.

What if I leave it for a couple of days to think about things?

As above, this will help you determine whether your midwife or doctor is open to finding a solution that meets your hopes for your birth as well as their judgement about what the 'best' course of action is. Although professionals have knowledge about pregnancy and birth in general, you are the expert on your body and your baby, although this is not often acknowledged in a meaningful way within the maternity services.

At the very least, even if you are told you need an immediate induction for what you consider to be a good reason, you might like to take a walk or find a place to sit for a few minutes outside the hospital with whoever is with you in order to think about the decision and get used to the idea. If there are aspects of the induction process you want to know more about, this is the time to ask questions and discuss it further. You may find things move quite quickly after this, and it may be more difficult to stop the process and/or ask questions later on.

It is not the law!

Recently, AIMS was contacted by a woman who was told she had to be induced 'because it was the law'. Because of this, she agreed to induction (which was recommended because her waters had broken more than 24 hours previously) and went on to have what she felt was a very traumatic birth. She was apparently told by a health professional that 'We have to induce you 24 hours after rupture of membranes. It's the law'.

Please be aware that there are no laws that state what a pregnant woman must or must not do. AIMS is very concerned about this issue and we want to assure you that this should not happen. In fact, this is such a serious breach of professional responsibility that any practitioner saying such a thing should be reported to their professional body. Any woman who is threatened in any way or told something of this nature is welcome to contact AIMS for information and support and may find it useful to contact a local Supervisor of Midwives. AIMS is happy to contact Supervisors of Midwives if, for any reason, the woman would prefer this.

How to contact a Supervisor of Midwives

There is always a Supervisor of Midwives on duty. She is there to support women and midwives and can be contacted any time.

Probably the easiest way to do this is to call your local hospital and ask for the contact details of a Supervisor of Midwives; a large hospital will have several Supervisors of Midwives.

More information on how to contact a Supervisor of Midwives is available here:
www.nmc-uk.org/patients-public/Women-and-families/How-supervisors-of-midwives-can-help-you/.

You might also want to ask for the name and contact details of the Head of Midwifery (who may also be a Supervisor).

If you need further advice or help with finding out about your rights or how to make a complaint, you can contact AIMS or download a copy of Making a complaint about maternity care from the AIMS website.

Part Three

Induction – The Evidence

This part of the book looks at the research evidence relating to different questions about induction of labour. It is designed to be used in conjunction with the explanations of different aspects of induction of labour in Part One.

Before we look at any specific questions, though, I would like to say a bit more about the way in which different people (including midwives, doctors, researchers and others) take different attitudes to childbirth in general and induction of labour in particular, and what this means in relation to the way they interpret the research evidence. Because, no matter how strongly people protest otherwise, it is entirely possible for two reasonable people (or, in the case of the guidelines developed by professional bodies or national organisations, groups of people) to look at the same research evidence and draw different conclusions from it.

This could be seen as a problem in the sense that it means that there is no one right way of looking at a situation or question, and in turn means we each have to decide what we think and feel about something. (Of course some people prefer to decide not to decide and want their health professionals to decide, which is fine too. In such situations the professionals are likely to choose the 'do as much as possible' approach because, quite understandably, they want to be able to say, 'We did everything we could'.) But I think it can be helpful to understand that two people, who both seem very nice and reasonable and caring, can have really different viewpoints.

There are several reasons that can explain why people might draw different conclusions from the same evidence, but I will limit myself to briefly explaining the three that I think are the most important:

1. Different people have different beliefs about birth. Some see it as a very natural journey or process and feel it is best to interfere as little as possible. They don't want to use technology or drugs unless it is truly necessary. Others focus more on the possible risks and think it is best to take as many precautions as possible, even if some of the risks are very rare and the precautions taken may disrupt the natural process. They may argue that we live in a modern world and should take advantage of the things that we have learned. These different approaches can lead to differing views about topics such as induction, and people are often more likely to see their own view reflected in the research that they read than to see another view.

2. When the difference between different groups (for example the outcomes of women who had their labour induced at 41 weeks of pregnancy compared with women who awaited spontaneous labour) are so slight, the researcher and the reader have more leeway to decide for themselves what this means. I once analysed a review of 10 studies of induction of labour whose results all showed no difference between the outcomes of the women who were induced and the women who waited for spontaneous labour. Yet in the text of the conclusions of the papers that had presented those results, five had said that there was no difference in the numbers of babies who died so it was up to the clinician or woman, three said there was no difference so it was better not to interfere, and

two said there was no difference so we may as well carry on inducing everybody when they reach 41 weeks!

3. Finally, people may draw different conclusions because they look more or less closely at the way in which the researchers carried out their study. No research study is perfect, but some studies are more liable to be biased (whether accidentally or otherwise) than others. Sometimes, the reason that two people disagree about the value or meaning of the results of a research study is because one is concerned that the study may be biased and that this has influenced the results.

Now that I have said that, it will probably not surprise you if I also suggest that, just because a guideline is approved by a professional or national body, it does not mean that it is the best or only view on the subject. This is partly because guidelines are written for people who are caring for whole populations of women who are very different from each other. However, individual women need to make a decision about what is best for them as an individual.

The latest UK guidelines that we can draw upon are the NICE (2008) guidelines and the update that was issued in 2013. I do think it is useful to include details of what the guidance says because it can help to make clear what the basis for professional suggestions might be. Sometimes this will explain why someone is suggesting a particular course of action. Knowing what the guidelines suggest can be helpful, for instance, if a professional is recommending a course of action that is different from what the guidelines suggest.

There are times in this book where I will tell you what the national guidelines say about induction but also offer a different perspective on the same evidence.

No matter whether we are talking about the contents of guidelines or the perspective of an individual midwife or doctor, the existence of different perspectives can be confusing. I will try to offer some examples of these when we look at the evidence on the following pages, but I hope that the above explanation might help make a bit more sense of what can be a really confusing situation.

I think the take-home message from this is: be aware that you may talk to health professionals or read guidelines written by people who have read the same research studies and take an entirely different view of them. This doesn't necessarily mean that one person is right and the other wrong. It does mean that you need to make the decision that is right for you as an individual within the context of your own life, beliefs and family. For more on this please see the AIMS booklet *What's Right For Me?*

Finally, to save me from writing it at the end of every section, there is a significant omission in the data that we are going to discuss. There is an almost complete lack of good research that considers what women think, looks at long-term effects and looks at the possible psychological outcomes of these interventions. The focus is almost always on short-term physical outcomes. I hear about the long-term and psychological effects of childbirth almost every time I sit next to a woman on a train or aeroplane who asks me what I do for a living, and (as I imagine many people reading this already know), no matter whether the memories are positive, negative or both, they last forever.

A few of the studies discussed in the following pages have asked women what they think, but the methods used are generally not very likely to give reliable results. If you had had a bad experience and were asked about your care by a uniformed member of staff before you were discharged from hospital, do you think you would be completely honest in every situation? In 1984, an important study by Porter and MacIntyre showed that pregnant women seemed to assume that whatever they had experienced was the best possible arrangement and to be negative about other possibilities until they had experienced them. These results were confirmed nearly twenty years later by van Teijlingen et al (2003), who showed that people tend to value the status quo mire highly than things of which they have no experience, which further confirmed that such studies are not a good way of finding out what women really think. Again, we would encourage you to visit www.aims.org.uk/birthStories to read women's stories.

When do the NICE guidelines recommend NOT inducing?

Every version of the national guidance to date has included a list of situations in which induction of labour is not considered appropriate. Some of these situations are included because, in the past, some practitioners have seen them as reasons for induction and the team who wrote the guidance is making clear that these situations are not in themselves reasons to induce labour. It is also important to remember that there are sometimes exceptions to these general rules.

Breech baby: Induction of labour is not generally recommended when a baby is in the breech position, unless delivery is indicated and the woman declines caesarean section. In this case, the risks must be discussed. Midwives who attend breech births are very concerned about the potential risks of induction where the baby is breech and the AIMS booklet *Breech Birth - What are my options?* contains more information about this.

Fast labour: Induction is also not recommended in an attempt to avoid precipitate birth; that is, when a woman has had a previous fast labour and given birth before a health professional can arrive.

Small baby: Induction is not recommended when there is fetal growth restriction; that is, the baby is thought to be not growing appropriately.

Large baby: In the absence of other indications (which may change things), induction is not recommended in situations where a healthcare professional suspects that a baby is large for gestational age (fetal macrosomia). It is important to note in relation to this and the above point that we have no really accurate way of predicting the baby's size.

Maternally requested induction

Induction is also not generally recommended at maternal request, and the NICE (2008) guidelines state this far more clearly than did the previous guidelines (RCOG 2001). It is, however, acknowledged that sometimes exceptional circumstances apply, such as when a woman's partner is being posted abroad. It is perhaps inevitable that, because some doctors tend to favour intervention in labour rather than natural birth, some women who request induction find that this is seen as a 'good choice' by their doctor and have no problem achieving their aim. Others, however, find that it can be just as hard to persuade a health professional that you want or need to be induced as it is to persuade a health professional that you don't want or need to be induced! If this is your experience, AIMS may be able to help and support you. The information in part Two may also be useful in enabling you to be more informed about the process of induction so that you can discuss your views effectively with the people who are caring for you.

Induction after a baby has died

In the very sad event that a baby dies before labour begins, NICE (2008) recommends that (as well as lots of support, information and help) – as long as the woman is physically well, her waters have not broken and she is not bleeding – health professionals should offer the choice of immediate induction of labour or expectant management (which means waiting for spontaneous labour while they keep an eye on the woman's health and monitor the situation). There is no evidence which suggests that automatically inducing labour is beneficial on a physical level. Some women feel that they would prefer to wait and allow their labour to start spontaneously, while others may feel more comfortable with having their labour induced quickly.

Some of the risks of induction to babies sadly become irrelevant in this situation, although there are still risks for the mother herself. For this reason, if a woman's waters have broken or if there is infection or bleeding, induction is more likely to be recommended because these situations carry an increased risk of infection to the woman, which can sometimes become serious quickly. However, a more straightforward labour and birth may have a positive effect on the woman's ability to conceive, carry and birth any subsequent babies.

If you are facing this decision, you may wish to reconsider any birth plan you have made in the light of the situation. For instance, some women decide that they would prefer to labour and give birth in their own homes, even though they had previously planned to give birth in hospital. Others might find that their feelings about whether or not they would choose pain relief change in this situation. It may be well worth taking a little time to think about how you feel about your options before you rush into any decisions, and your health professionals should be sensitive and respectful of this.

AIMS is always willing to talk to women who need support. SANDS, the stillbirth and neonatal death charity, also exists to support anyone affected by such issues, and its website can be found at www.uk-sands.org.

Induction after previous caesarean section

The current UK NICE guidance (2008) suggests that, in the event that a professional caring for a woman who has had a previous caesarean section has a good reason to recommend early delivery rather than awaiting spontaneous labour, the woman may be offered induction of labour with prostaglandin, a repeat caesarean section or expectant management on an individual basis. The guidelines are clear that the woman's circumstances and wishes should be taken into account. Women should be informed of the increased risks with induction of labour after a caesarean section, including the increased risk of the need for emergency caesarean section and the increased risk of uterine rupture.

The guideline is only talking about where the woman is experiencing a problem or situation where delivery is specifically indicated. It does not say that all women who have had a previous caesarean section should be offered induction. Indeed, as the guideline notes, women who have had a previous caesarean section face increased risks if they have an induction. With that in mind, it is important to be clear about why someone is suggesting that delivery is warranted. This might lead you to look elsewhere in the book, for instance at the section on prolonged pregnancy or maternal age. As the guideline suggests, there are three main options, which are:

- induction;

- caesarean section;

- waiting, perhaps with further monitoring.

If you face this decision (and even if you have not had a previous caesarean section), don't forget that choosing the third option does not mean you have to wait for as long as labour takes. You can choose to wait 24 hours and come back tomorrow, to wait 48 or 72 hours and come back over the weekend, to go home and wait for your partner to come home to discuss it and then return later that day … the possibilities are often greater than people realise in the moment when they face the decision.

Induction of labour in women with diabetes

There are two types of women who might consider that the information under this heading concerns them: women who have insulin-dependent diabetes and women who develop so-called gestational diabetes in pregnancy. Unfortunately, both of these areas are, for slightly different reasons, outside the scope of this book, but I want to try to offer brief explanations of why this is, and some suggestions of things to consider.

I will consider the latter group first: women who have gestational diabetes. I wrote 'so-called' gestational diabetes in the paragraph above because some midwives and doctors question whether this is even a real condition. I know of women who have been told that they need to be induced because they have gestational diabetes, but there is a real lack of consistency in the research in this area, partly because different researchers use different definitions, tests and protocols. I would like to reiterate at this point that the NICE (2008) guidance is clear that induction is not indicated simply because it is thought that the baby may be large (macrosomic).

Women who have insulin-dependent diabetes (IDD) are at more risk of having poorer outcomes because of the needs that their condition creates and the impact that it can have on babies. This doesn't mean they have to give up all choice; for example, I know of women with really well-controlled insulin-dependent diabetes who have had waterbirths and even birthed at home, but it would not be fair to women in this group to try and gloss over the greater challenges that they face. Unfortunately, the question of whether and when induction is warranted in women who have IDD is too complex and uncertain to be covered in this book, and the NICE (2008) guidance does not cover this area. I hope, however, that some of the information and questions in other sections will be helpful guides to the kind of conversations that you might have with your caregivers about your individual circumstances.

Induction in twin (or more!) pregnancies

This is another area that is not covered by the NICE (2008) guideline or in this book. As the RCOG (2001) guideline noted, it is not possible to make recommendations for or against induction in twin or multiple (more babies) pregnancy because there is not enough evidence to suggest that this is beneficial. The rate of perinatal (around the time of birth) mortality is higher with multiples than with single babies, but this does not automatically mean there is any benefit to be gained from induction of labour. Twin births are more likely to be early than late, and any number of babies more than this almost certainly so, and the combination of this and the current medical trend for recommending caesarean section for twin or multiple births means that the need to consider induction doesn't arise as often for women who are pregnant with more than one baby.

Induction for other obstetric or medical reasons

This seems a good point to take stock and summarise where we are at so far, because we have looked at a number of situations that can be fairly clearly defined (even if the evidence isn't). Next I will cover what I have come to call the 'big three' induction decisions, but that will still leave quite a few grey areas. These grey areas concern situations in which a woman might be told that induction is warranted in her particular case, for example where she has a condition such as pre-eclampsia, obstetric cholestasis, antibody problems or a disease that the woman has which cannot be treated until the baby is born.

No two people ever experience a disease or problem in exactly the same way, and this is one reason why there are no hard and fast rules (and often no research studies) that can help with decision-making. None of these situations are hard and fast; if they were common, or if there were clear indications for induction of labour that were either supported by evidence or of such concern that they featured in the national guidance, then they would have been discussed under their own heading. But, again, I hope that the various question lists elsewhere in this book might help you explore why induction is being offered in your circumstances.

In particular, you might want to ask whether it is routine to induce somebody in your situation or whether there are specific indications which apply to you. You could also ask whoever is recommending induction of labour to talk you through the evidence that is underpinning their decision.

Some women ask for copies of or links to relevant papers so they can look at the evidence themselves. Gaining as much information as you can about why induction is being suggested will enable you to go and get further information (if you want to) so that you are well informed about the most recent information relating to your situation. Remember that not all information is equally valid; sometimes you need to take a careful look at whether it is based on accurate data. Also, as we have discussed, there are some huge areas of uncertainty and it may boil down to what you think and believe – which is why it can be quite helpful to try and find out whether the person recommending induction generally thinks and believes the same things as you. Finally, AIMS is always here if you need support or information or if you feel it would be useful to talk through the decision or the issues with someone who is not involved.

Induction for prolonged pregnancy

Being 'overdue' (or 'post-dates', or having a 'prolonged' pregnancy) is the most common reason given to women to justify an induction of labour. I have put each of these terms in quotation marks in this paragraph because they are often used in ways that are contentious and it may be important to think about what people are implying when they use them. For instance, can we really know that a particular pregnancy is prolonged or a particular baby is overdue? The pregnancy might have been a bit longer than average, and the baby's birthday on the later side of normal in relation to the estimated due date, but the human idea of normal includes a range of possibilities. It is important to remember that longer (or shorter) can be really, really normal and healthy for some women and babies. Also, because the word 'term' means anytime between 37 and 42 completed weeks of pregnancy, saying that a pregnancy is 'post-term' when the woman is only 41 weeks pregnant is inaccurate.

Although the NICE guideline states that a prolonged pregnancy is a pregnancy that lasts beyond 42 weeks, the exact timing of when a baby is deemed to be overdue seems to differ according to where you live, which research studies underpin local policy and what the local obstetricians think. Whereas even a few years ago the majority of women could expect their pregnancy to continue for up to 42 weeks before they needed to consider whether or not they wanted induction, many areas now routinely offer induction of labour from 41 weeks of pregnancy. (Some people justify this by saying that it can take a couple of days before the baby will actually be born, so it is better to start early, while others feel it is simply increasing the induction rate without offering any benefit.)

The prevalence of induction means that it is quite hard to know how many women would still be pregnant at different points in the absence of induction of labour, but we can estimate from various documents and statistics that 5 - 10 per cent of all women are still pregnant at the end of 42 weeks (NICE 2008) and that more than one in five women has their labour induced for being 'overdue'.

NICE recommendations on prevention of prolonged pregnancy are that:

- *Women with uncomplicated pregnancies should be given every opportunity to go into spontaneous labour.*

- *Women with uncomplicated pregnancies should usually be offered induction of labour between 41+0 and 42+0 weeks to avoid the risks of prolonged pregnancy. The exact timing should take into account the woman's preferences and local circumstances.*

- *If a woman chooses not to have induction of labour, her decision should be respected. Healthcare professionals should discuss the woman's care with her from then on.*

- *From 42 weeks, women who decline induction of labour should be offered increased antenatal monitoring consisting of at least twice-weekly cardiotocography and ultrasound estimation of maximum amniotic pool depth (NICE 2008: 10).*

But what are the risks that induction of labour seeks to avoid? Many people have come to believe that pregnancy can become dangerous beyond a certain point in time and that induction of labour can improve outcomes, but the evidence is not clear-cut. We will look more at this below but, because it is a crucial element of this area, I will first look at how the due date is calculated and what implications this might have for decisions about induction of labour.

Dating pregnancy

'It is also imperative that the most accurate information is obtained concerning the gestational age of the pregnancy.' (NICE 2008: 2)

Only about 5 per cent of babies arrive on their due date (Khambalia et al 2013) and yet this date has long been perceived as a critical piece of information by midwives and doctors (Anderson 2000), and often by women themselves. If women choose to have any antenatal screening tests, the due date can affect when these are carried out (which can then affect how accurate they are) and, on a more practical level, it enables families to plan for the arrival of their new baby. There are three basic ways of estimating a due date:

Calculating from the woman's last menstrual period

While both ancient Hindu and Roman cultures recognised that pregnancy lasted around nine months (Saunders and Paterson 1991), it was Aristotle who first documented the average length of pregnancy as being ten lunar months, which is widely accepted as being 280 days (Rosser 2000). This period of time was later used as the basis for Naegele's rule, a rule of thumb that calculates the baby's due date by adding seven days and nine months to the first day of a woman's last menstrual period before she became pregnant.

If you work this out with a few random dates, you will see that the two are not exactly aligned – this is mainly because the months of the year vary a bit in length – and most of the obstetric calculators used today give a due date somewhere between Naegele's rule and

280 days. This, in combination with an understanding of the very real impact that even a few days' difference in the due date can make to women, is one of the reasons why midwife Tricia Anderson (2000) advised midwives to exercise caution when using what she called whirly wheel calculators to calculate a woman's due date and her current gestation at each antenatal visit. If a midwife or doctor uses one of these during an antenatal visit and tells you that you are a slightly different number of weeks and days pregnant from what you thought, this is almost certainly why.

Naegele's rule has never been substantiated by research. Furthermore, a slow but steady stream of research and articles has challenged the assumptions that (a) pregnancy lasts for 280 days and (b) the same calculation should be used for everyone. In the 1990s, Mittendorf et al (1990, 1993) carried out several related studies showing that pregnancy length was longer than Naegele's rule suggests and that it varied according to characteristics such as height, ethnicity and parity (whether a woman has had babies before). Mittendorf's research also uncovered evidence that pregnancy length was affected by the length of a woman's mother's and grandmother's pregnancies and that there were genetic and ethnic differences. My own research uncovered many examples and stories of this occurring in practice, and I also believe that there are influences from the baby's father. One of my colleagues who read an early draft of this book shared her family's example of this with me. She had four pregnancies where she did not go into labour before 43 weeks. She was herself born before 40 weeks but her husband was born at 44 weeks and his brother induced at 43 weeks. We have also long known that the lengths of women's menstrual cycles can vary and the calculators in use assume that all women have a menstrual cycle lasting 28 days. All of these assumptions can lead to a woman's due date being inaccurate by several days.

In 2013, Jukic et al used urine samples to calculate exactly when conception took place and again showed that the average length of pregnancy was longer than we usually allow for. I found several papers that had proposed this in different ways (Wickham 2010, 2011), but they have all but been ignored in practice. I also found that holistic midwives who were practising outside the system of maternity care in their country (such as independent midwives in the UK) were well aware of this evidence and were using it to individualise the calculation of the due date, but I cannot find any evidence that it has been taken into account in mainstream practice or in the guidelines that underpin this. Most practitioners still use Naegele's rule.

Calculating from a known conception date

A variation on the above method involves performing the same kind of calculation but using the date of conception rather than the date of the last menstrual period. Although the questions about whether we are using an appropriate length of pregnancy and whether we need to take individual variation into account still apply, using the conception date may make the date slightly more accurate than the last menstrual period (LMP) date. Using the LMP date relies on an assumption that the woman's last period started a certain number of days before conception, and in reality there is variation in this between different women too.

However, until relatively recently, even though many women believed that they knew exactly when they conceived, they were not always believed by health professionals. Where conception occurs naturally, this is often still the case. The thing that has changed in recent years is the number of women who use assisted reproductive technologies (ARTs), and the doctors performing these are believed, so this is one instance when this date might be used, but it will still generally be used together with the assumption that pregnancy lasts for 280 days.

Ultrasound

The NICE guidance states that:

'In most instances, there will be reliable menstrual data supported by evidence from an ultrasound examination made in the early weeks of pregnancy and, indeed, nowadays the information from the latter source will take precedence from the clinician's perspective even though many women are clear about their own due dates.' (NICE 2008: 2)

Some interpreters of the research evidence would disagree that ultrasound is a more reliable means of dating pregnancy. Most of the studies that have been set up to evaluate ultrasound dating have generally looked at it in comparison with Naegele's rule and, as we already know that this is not very accurate, it seems ill-advised that this is the benchmark against which the accuracy of ultrasound has been measured! There are a number of other problems with the studies that have evaluated ultrasound dating. In several, women and their midwives knew what the predicted due dates were, so this may have influenced when the women actually gave birth. It is probably stating the obvious to say that babies come in a range of different sizes, yet this variation in size between babies can still result in a lot of potential mistakes when ultrasound is used to calculate due date. This has been pointed out for years (such as by Moore et al in 1991), but ultrasound practitioners and researchers have not really addressed this fundamental issue.

Some medical reviewers (Whitworth et al 2010) suggest that early pregnancy ultrasound is associated with a reduced incidence of post-term pregnancy. This means that most women are offered dating scans at early antenatal visits. However, work by Khambalia et al (2013) showed that there were no meaningful differences between the prediction of date of birth by ultrasound scan date and menstrual dating. They expressed concerns about the risks of early dating scans and concluded that a scan before or at 10 weeks is unnecessary if the LMP date is reliable. Consumer organisations such as AIMS have also spent years voicing concerns about the safety of ultrasound, which is not proven to be the safe intervention that many people assume it to be (Robinson 2000, Beech 2004). There is almost a complete lack of research into the risks of this technology, but what little research has been done tells us that ultrasound does cause problems, which is worrying given that ultrasound is so readily accepted that many women sign up to have expensive three or four dimensional scans, which expose their baby to ultrasound for even longer.

What to do?

Back in 1991, Stronge and Rasmussen argued that midwives and doctors should admit that predicting a due date is no more accurate than forecasting weather, and in the twenty or so years that have passed since their words were published, our predictions have not really improved. Indeed, all but a handful of people have systematically ignored the evidence that has proposed ways in which we could improve our calculations of the due date for individual women. Certainly there is evidence to suggest that length of pregnancy is based on many factors, including the father's genetics (Lie et al 2006) and the baby herself.

Despite their not taking into account the evidence around the need for individualisation, the NICE (2008: 2) guidelines state that 'Where evidence from these sources is lacking and the gestational age is in doubt, extra care should be taken in assessing the balance of risks [of induction for prolonged pregnancy].' This is an important acknowledgement of the fact that, if the due date is inaccurate and induction of labour is carried out, the baby can be born too early. It is worrying that scan dates are given precedence over women's dates even though scans can predict a date too early or too late due to variations in growth rates.

You and your baby are the people who are going to be most affected by the way your due date is calculated. With that in mind, you might want to consider the following:

- If you think that a due date you have been given at the beginning of pregnancy is incorrect, discuss this with your midwife or doctor sooner rather than later, as it could have serious repercussions later in your pregnancy. It is easier to negotiate those changes early in pregnancy than when you are considered to be 41 weeks pregnant by an inaccurate due date and are in the middle of a conversation with someone who is suggesting induction. But, if you find that someone won't change your due date for some reason, ask them to record your feelings about this in your notes, next to where they have written the due date. Or, if you carry or have access to your own notes in which you can write, you can make such a note yourself.

- If your menstrual cycle is longer or shorter than 28 days, or if your last period was unusual, this may cause the calculation of the due date to be inaccurate. Let your midwife know that you want this taken into account when your due date is calculated. Midwives often ask if your last period was a normal period. If it wasn't, tell them that and then ask whether and how they will take that into account when calculating the due date.

- If you are sure of your menstrual dates, think carefully before you accept that an ultrasound date is more accurate. You may simply have a baby who is, at the moment, a bit bigger or smaller than average.

- If you are certain of and happy with your due date and concerned about whether, if you have a scan, this may be changed, negotiate this beforehand. The more women ask about this, the more professionals will take it into account.

- If you have concerns about your due date calculation which you feel are not being heard, do not hesitate to contact a Supervisor of Midwives. Many professionals feel bound to follow the hospital rules around this, but these are not set in stone and, because the implications of the due date are so enormous (and because you may not feel up to the challenge or debate when you are heavily pregnant and tired), it is worth doing what you can to ensure that it is right at the outset. You can always contact AIMS for support and information if you need to.

- If you are reading this and not yet pregnant, or if you are planning to have more babies in the future, it is worth thinking about keeping charts of your menstrual cycle, so you have information about your own body which can help you and your midwife work out your due date. You can even get phone apps that pretty much do it for you!

Introducing the prolonged pregnancy debate

Because the research in this area is complex, I would like to begin this section with a summary of what I tell women about prolonged pregnancy. Then I will spend the next few pages explaining the research findings that underpin my summary.

Although the vast majority of pregnancies have very happy endings, pregnancy never comes with a guarantee that every baby will be born alive and well. We have long known that babies who are born prematurely are not as likely to survive, and there is some statistical evidence showing that babies who are born very late in pregnancy may also be less likely to survive. This is why induction is recommended for prolonged pregnancy.

However, the increased risk comes later than most people think, is less than most people think and cannot necessarily be prevented by induction of labour. Induction of labour also carries risks to the baby and the woman, so the decision is not nearly as clear-cut as most people think.

There is increasing and global agreement that routine induction, especially for prolonged pregnancy, is problematic:

- Although the World Health Organisation (2011) guidelines recommend induction of labour for women who are known with certainty to have reached 41 weeks of pregnancy, they state that the quality of evidence for this recommendation is low and the strength of the evidence is weak.

- Glantz noted that, in the US, where many of the studies relating to this question were carried out, *'labour induction and cesarean section rates have doubled over the past three decades without proportional improvement in perinatal outcome.'* (Glantz 2012: 289)

- A Canadian analysis of data gathered from 1,601,253 (yes, over one and a half million!) women's medical records *'confirmed that induction of labor is associated with higher rates of specific severe maternal morbidity among women without documented pregnancy complications, especially at 38 and 39 weeks' gestation, although all rate differences were small and the numbers needed to demonstrate harm were large. Nevertheless, these serious risks must be balanced against potential benefits whenever the decision to induce labor is considered.'* (Liu et al 2013: 209.e1)

- In the UK, the Database of Uncertainties about the Effects of Treatments (DUETs – www.library.nhs.uk/duets/) is a resource which highlights areas where evidence about the effects of treatments is lacking. The July 2013 NICE Evidence Update, which considers whether new evidence should lead to changes in the recommendations, added *'induction of labour for improving outcomes at or beyond term'* to the database because it was identified as an area in which uncertainties exist.

What is normal?

Because induction of labour has been a common feature of maternity care for many years, it is incredibly difficult to know how many women would still be pregnant at any given point of pregnancy in a world without medical induction. But one study that might help to put the following sections into context was conducted by Heimstad et al (2008) in Norway. In showing just how many women are affected by the policy of inducing labour at different points, we can also take from this the fact that it is really normal for some women to have a pregnancy that lasts longer than average.

- If all of the women whose pregnancies reached 41 weeks were offered induction, 240 women would be offered induction for every 1000 pregnant women. This means that nearly one in four women is still pregnant by the end of 41 weeks of pregnancy. (Given that induction of labour is routinely recommended at or around 41 weeks in some areas, this explains why the induction rate is so high.)

- If women were instead offered induction only when their pregnancy reached 42 weeks, 90 out of 1000 women would be offered induction. So just under one in ten women are still pregnant by the time they reach 42 weeks.

- If women were offered induction only if their pregnancy reached 43 weeks, only four per 1000 women would be offered induction. So, if they decided to wait, only one in 250 women would still be pregnant by the end of 43 weeks.

Is prolonged pregnancy risky?

I said above that the increased risk comes later than most people think, is less than most people think and cannot necessarily be prevented by induction of labour. I would like to explain this a bit more now, in relation to the research findings, and also to show you how some of the uncertainties and confusions in this area have led to the current situation.

For example, one of the reasons this area is confusing is that different countries, hospitals, doctors and midwives have different cut-off points as to when they consider that pregnancy has continued to the point that it is better to offer induction. If you re-read the first bullet point on page 76, you will see I wrote that the World Health Organisation (2011) recommends induction for women who are known to have reached 41 weeks of pregnancy. But didn't I say on page 66 that a normal term pregnancy could last up to 42 weeks?

There are a number of reasons for this discrepancy. Where people are making guidelines for whole populations of women, they tend to err on the side of caution. If, say, you wanted to make sure that every woman was offered the chance to have her baby born by the time her pregnancy had reached 42 weeks, then you would need to take a few things into account. It usually takes a day or two between the first dose of prostaglandin and the arrival of the baby, so if you want the baby born by 42 weeks, then you need to start induction at 41 weeks and 5 days. But what if the labour ward is busy and you have to wait for a bed? Best give it an extra couple of days' leeway, just in case, so that takes us to an induction date of, say, 41 weeks and 3 days. Oh, but we don't like to start inductions on the weekend unless we really have to, because we have fewer staff available if caesarean sections are needed, so anyone who reaches that date on a Saturday might end up having their baby too late, so maybe it's best to say we'll offer induction to everybody at 41 weeks, and that way we can almost guarantee that every baby will be born by 42 weeks of pregnancy…

I probably don't need to spell out the implications of this. Far more women get induced than might be necessary because (as is so often the case) we are applying the worst-case scenario to everybody. This problem partly occurs because maternity services have been centralised and it is now unusual for women to have one midwife taking care of them, which means that policies have to ensure that women do not 'fall between the cracks'.

But there is another important question here. Is it really the case that there is a significant difference in risk for babies born at 41 weeks and 6 days and babies born at 42 weeks? Sadly, stillbirth can and does happen at all stages of pregnancy, and many stillbirths cannot be prevented. The induction for post-term policies seem to imply that something terrible happens on the stroke of midnight at 42 weeks, but is this really the case?

In answering this question, I would first like to remind you that, in the section on dating pregnancy on page 68, we saw how this is not an exact science and that there is considerable variation between women. So if it is normal that some women naturally have longer pregnancies than others, then surely we can't know that there is an exact time, which is the same for everybody, when problems would occur if the baby hasn't been born?

The idea that something terrible will happen if a woman remains pregnant for a moment longer than 42 weeks just isn't true. I would like to quote my friend and colleague Julie Frohlich here. Julie is a consultant midwife who has a lot of experience supporting women making decisions in this and many other areas, and she tells women that *'the baby does not turn into a pumpkin on the stroke of 42 weeks'.*

My own research with holistic midwives (Wickham 2009, 2010, 2011) revealed that many of us say the same kind of thing. This is because, although there is a slight increase in risk if a pregnancy lasts for more than 42 weeks, it is nowhere near as big an increase as the induction policies might imply, and there is certainly nothing drastic that happens overnight between 41 weeks and 6 days and 42 weeks of pregnancy. There is no clear dividing line, no clock chime that marks a clear point between everything being OK one day and risk-laden the next. The idea that the placenta gets worn out in late pregnancy is also a very unhelpful one, as, while some women do have problems, there is no evidence that this is related to length of pregnancy. In fact, when we (mis)place our trust in a date-based policy which says that we should routinely offer induction at 41-42 weeks, we are not only subjecting a lot of women and babies to unnecessary induction, we are probably also not paying enough attention to picking up the signals from babies who actually need help before 41 weeks. We might well have better outcomes if we gave individualised care rather than acting as if every woman and baby were the same.

In addition, the actual increase in risk is smaller than some people believe, and, while the numbers are complex, many people consider that the difference only really becomes significant once a woman has been pregnant for 43 weeks. For the past few years, the reference most commonly used in the UK documents was a paper by Hilder et al, published in 1998, which showed that the rate of perinatal death is at its lowest at about one in a thousand at 41 weeks, rising to about two in a thousand from 42 weeks. It was on the basis of this data that it was proposed that routinely offering induction of labour between 41 and 42 weeks might prevent the death of those additional one in a thousand babies. (Below, we will look at whether this worked). Some women were told that the risk to their baby doubled at this time, but I hope you can see from these figures that, while this statement was technically accurate, it might not have been the clearest way of discussing the situation with women.

The numbers change drastically depending on what you measure and how you measure it. They change according to whether you divide the number of babies who die in each week by all of the babies who were born in that week (which most people now agree isn't the best way of doing it) or by all the babies who remain unborn. Then what do we do about babies who are known to have a problem which has nothing to do with length of pregnancy or induction of labour? We can see this in another study which was published in the British Medical Journal by Cotzias et al in 1999, and which looked at unexplained stillbirth in each week of pregnancy in relation to the number of ongoing pregnancies. In this study:

The risk of an unexplained stillbirth at 35 weeks was 1 in 500
The risk of an unexplained stillbirth at 36 weeks was 1 in 556
The risk of an unexplained stillbirth at 37 weeks was 1 in 645
The risk of an unexplained stillbirth at 38 weeks was 1 in 730
The risk of an unexplained stillbirth at 39 weeks was 1 in 840
The risk of an unexplained stillbirth at 40 weeks was 1 in 926
The risk of an unexplained stillbirth at 41 weeks was 1 in 826
The risk of an unexplained stillbirth at 42 weeks was 1 in 769
The risk of an unexplained stillbirth at 43 weeks was 1 in 633

The week in which women in this study were least likely to have an unexplained stillbirth was week 40, then weeks 39 and 41. If we look even more closely, we can see that the risk of an unexplained stillbirth at 42 weeks is actually less than the risk at 38 weeks. Yet 38 weeks is considered a normal and healthy time to have a baby. We don't routinely say to women who are 38 weeks pregnant, 'Gosh, you're 38 weeks pregnant now, so even though you were going to have your baby at home, you had better come into hospital and be induced instead!' Rather, (again assuming a level playing field in other regards) your midwife would be more likely to greet the news that you are labouring by saying something like, 'lucky you; you got to term, but now you don't have to wait for your due date!'

This is why I say that the risk occurs later than people think and is less than people think. It is also the case that it might not be preventable by induction. A Danish study by Olesen et al added further data in 2003. Like all studies of this kind, it relied on data from women who gave birth in previous years, which is important to know because policies and practices do change over time. This study also showed that there was a greater risk of death if babies were born later, but the data are not broken down by week of pregnancy and more than 12 per cent of the post-term births in this analysis occurred at or after 43 completed weeks of pregnancy. So the results aren't that helpful if we want to look at differences at, say, 41, 42 and 43 weeks of pregnancy.

But an important sentence in the Olesen et al (2003) paper is this one: *'Prolonged pregnancy may have causes that correlate with causes of the factors under study or prolonged pregnancy may be a response to already existing fetal disease'.*

In other words, it might not be the length of pregnancy itself that causes the problem. It may be that there exist one or more conditions which cause stillbirth AND prolonged pregnancy, and if this is the case then induction of labour might not make a difference to the outcome. But there are other elements of that question that we can consider as well, so let's look at those.

Does induction for prolonged pregnancy reduce risk?

In the section above, I have argued that the risk isn't as great as many people believe, but we can also consider the question of whether induction is beneficial from another angle. What can we learn from the research studies that compare women who are induced at a certain stage of pregnancy with women who remain pregnant?

It probably won't surprise you to read that these studies aren't perfect either. There are a number of ways in which their results may be biased, and Gülmezoglu et al (2012), who authored the Cochrane review in this area, showed that all of the included studies were at a high risk of bias because (inevitably) both the participating women and their caregivers knew whether or not they were being induced. Their analysis of the possible different types of bias in each of the studies showed that most of the studies were at moderate risk of bias. This is important, because it means the results may not be reliable, and we need to analyse what they mean carefully.

All of the studies, for example, were at high risk of bias due to lack of blinding of participants and personnel. In research, it is always considered better if people are 'blind' to whether they are getting the real treatment or the placebo. This is because of the placebo effect – when an outcome is different (either better or worse) because people expect that it will be different and so subconsciously and unintentionally influence it. Blinding is easy when you are doing a trial involving pills: you ask the hospital pharmacy to make some sugar pills that look and taste like the real pills, and then you put them into identical bottles. But it is impossible to use blinding in research evaluating the onset of labour, because women and their carers know exactly what is happening and which group they are in. This means, however, that some outcomes might have been subconsciously influenced by people's previous views of induction or non-induction.

For instance, a midwife or doctor who is uncomfortable with waiting for spontaneous labour might subconsciously expect the baby to be less well after birth, and this might affect the Apgar score which they give as a measure of the baby's well-being after birth. Or, as we think might have happened in one study (Hannah et al 1992), someone who was uncomfortable with not inducing women at 41 weeks might be more likely to suggest a caesarean section sooner in the women who had waited for spontaneous labour. This can falsely make it look as if caesarean section is less likely after induction, whereas in most of the other studies, and in the experience of many midwives and doctors, the opposite is the case.

Overall, the review suggested that induction of labour to avoid prolonged pregnancy may be associated with fewer perinatal deaths than expectant management. It also, possibly because of the inclusion of the flawed study mentioned above, suggested that induction reduces the caesarean section rate, but this finding is very debatable, as above, and has not been incorporated into either the 2008 NICE guidance or the 2013 update. The authors of the review note that:

'the favourable results for caesarean births in the large Hannah 1992 trial have been questioned by some authors. They have pointed out that the women who were induced in the policy of induction group (66% of this group) may have had a more effective cervical ripening regimen than the women who were induced in the expectant management group (33% of this group) and that more women in the expectant management group had a caesarean section for fetal distress (8.3% versus 5.7% in the induction group).' (Gülmezoglu et al 2012)

The Cochrane meta-analysis is not the only review of this area. Similar reviews were conducted by Wennerholm et al (2009), Sentilhes et al (2011) and Hussain et al (2011). Each of these reviews included – and excluded – different studies and, as a result, reached slightly different conclusions. But I think it is important to realise that all of the reviews of this area inevitably draw upon the results of more or less the same research studies. This means that, through no fault of the reviewers, the data that is used is based on the experiences of about 3000-3700 women who were allocated to be induced and 3000-3700 women who were allocated to waiting groups. The studies in the Cochrane review included one that was published in 1969, one in 1975, eight published in the 1980s, four in the 1990s and six published between 2000 and 2007. The practices experienced by the women who gave birth in the older trials will be very different from the practices employed nowadays.

The Cochrane review (Gülmezoglu et al 2012) goes on to point out that the UK (among other countries) only offers induction at 41 weeks (and I emphasise 'offers' because they are stressing that women do not have to consent to this) but our experience is that many women gain the impression that they will be putting their baby in danger if they do not consent to induction at this time. This fear is not supported by the data. Also, as Mandruzzato et al (2010) point out, the number of inductions needed to prevent one stillbirth is very high, at 416. So in order to prevent one stillbirth, you would need to 'intend to induce' at least 416 women's labours. I say 'intend to induce' because a small number of those women will go into labour or need a caesarean section before the induction begins, and it is impossible to remove those kinds of eventualities from the calculations. This means that those 416 (or more) women and their babies have to be exposed to the risks and downsides of induction itself, and to the risks and downsides of caesarean section in the case of the inductions that fail. How do we balance one set of risks against another?

Although these risks are discussed individually elsewhere, Baud et al (2013) compared overall adverse maternal and neonatal outcomes after elective (by women's choice) and medically indicated inductions of labour at term and found that, by comparison with labours that started spontaneously, induced labour increases the risk of caesarean or instrumental delivery, postpartum haemorrhage, prolonged maternal hospitalisation, having an Apgar score of less than 7 at 5 minutes of life and having an arterial umbilical cord pH of less than 7.1. The last of these indicates that the baby may have suffered from oxygen deprivation during the birth process. In an unrelated study, Yeh et al (2012) found that an arterial umbilical cord pH of less than 7.1 is associated with an increased risk of an adverse neurological outcome.

A few years ago, Menticoglou and Hall (2002) described the situation of inducing all women at or just after 41 weeks as *'nonsensus consensus'*. They argued that, while analysing the data one way (that is, the method used by the Cochrane reviewers) did seem to show that induction was better than waiting, there was another way of looking at the question. They took all of the data available at the time and considered whether each of the babies who died in the 'waiting' groups might have been saved by earlier induction of labour. They concluded that, when this question was considered and babies who could not have been saved by earlier induction of labour (for instance, those who had conditions that were incompatible with life) were removed from the analysis, there were no statistical differences between the outcomes of the babies in the induction group and the waiting group. Philip Hall, one of the authors of this paper, has sadly since died, and I do not know of an update to this paper that takes into account the latest (2012) version of the Cochrane review. But my assessment of this is that their main argument still stands. Even if there is a slight increase in perinatal mortality after a certain point in pregnancy, induction of labour would not necessarily save any babies. It does, however, lead to a number of other problems.

There is one last thing to bear in mind when making decisions about induction for so-called prolonged pregnancy. Even if a woman decides to await spontaneous labour and decline routine induction, she can still have monitoring if she wants and if at any point she and/or her doctor or midwife are worried, she can choose to be induced. In other words, this is not an all or nothing, now or never decision. It is quite reasonable for a woman to say, 'No, I do not want my labour to be induced at 41 weeks, but I would like an appointment at (say) 41 weeks and 5 days in order to talk about whether I may want to be induced at 42 weeks,' or, 'I do not want my labour to be induced at this point but I will let my midwife know if I change my mind'.

When women decide not to be automatically induced just because they have reached a certain date, they are likely to be offered monitoring to check on their baby. This may include more frequent checking of the baby's heartbeat and/or an ultrasound to measure the amount of water around the baby. Some women find this provides useful information in their decision-making, but it is important to remember that no screening test is totally accurate. This is another area where we need more research, and women who are more than 42 weeks pregnant will find that, because the majority of women are induced before they reach this point, we know very little about what the normal volume of fluid (or other things) should be at this stage of pregnancy.

Induction after the waters break

The amniotic sac, or bag of waters, that protects the baby in the uterus can break at any point before, during or at the end of the birth journey. For some women, this is the first sign that they are going into labour, and it will be followed soon afterwards by uterine contractions which get stronger until they give birth. Other women find that their waters break during their labour. Sometimes the membranes which contain the baby and the amniotic fluid can stay intact until the very end of labour, perhaps needing to be broken by the midwife just after the baby comes out, so he can breathe air.

Occasionally the waters might break a few weeks before the baby is expected to arrive, which can be a bit worrying. A few women's waters will break around the time the baby is expected to arrive but without any other signs of labour starting. In both of these cases, because there may be a risk of infection, induction may be discussed. We will look at each of these situations separately, because it makes a big difference whether the baby would be preterm or whether the woman is at or near the period we describe as 'term'. From 37 weeks onwards the baby would not be considered premature. In addition, some babies do seem to want to come a bit earlier than this but they are born healthy and well. As I am fond of saying, normal is a range, not a fixed point, and, as we saw on page 68, the dating of pregnancy is by no means an exact science.

When the waters break preterm and before labour

The NICE (2008) guidelines recommend that, if a woman has preterm prelabour rupture of membranes, induction of labour should not be carried out before 34 weeks unless there are additional obstetric indications (for example, infection or fetal compromise).

If a woman has preterm prelabour rupture of membranes after 34 weeks, the NICE guidelines recommend that the maternity team should discuss the following factors with her before a decision is made about whether to induce labour, using vaginal prostaglandin:

- risks to the woman (such as sepsis, possible need for caesarean section);

- risks to the baby (such as sepsis, problems relating to preterm birth);

- local availability of neonatal intensive care facilities.

This is because the studies that have looked at this area have found no evidence that infection, survival or sickness (in babies) rates are better if the woman chooses to be induced rather than waiting (Buchanan et al 2010). All of the trials have contained weaknesses and, even when their results are considered together, the numbers in them have been too small to detect meaningful differences in the rates of sickness and death. Induction does increase the caesarean section rate compared with waiting. The results of two more recent studies that were included in the NICE (2013) update (van der Ham et al 2012a, 2012b) did not provide any further insight.

It is important to be clear about what is being waited for and what waiting entails in this context, though. This is not the same as waiting for labour at term (say, like with prolonged pregnancy), where the women in the waiting groups might be at home and carry on as normal. Although women of course have the choice to decline, in this situation they would likely be offered ongoing tests and treatments, including antibiotics (to reduce the chance of infection), corticosteroids (to help the baby's lungs mature in case it is born prematurely) and/or admission to hospital, usually until the baby is born. In some of the studies, the researchers only waited until the women reached 37 weeks of pregnancy before labour was induced, and this is recommended in many areas.

The NICE guidelines also contain the following note:

'*Vaginal PGE2 [prostaglandin] has been used in UK practice for many years in women with ruptured membranes. However, the summary of product characteristics (SPCs) advise that in this situation, vaginal PGE2 is either not recommended or should be used with caution, depending on the preparation (gel, tablet or pessary). Healthcare professionals should refer to the individual SPCs before prescribing vaginal PGE2 for women with ruptured membranes, and informed consent should be obtained and documented.*' *(NICE 2013: 7)*

Again, I would like to refer you back to the section on dating pregnancy, as this might be an important issue if you are making a decision in this situation.

When the waters break at term and before labour

The NICE (2008) guidelines recommend that women with prelabour rupture of membranes at term (at or over 37 weeks) should be offered a choice of induction of labour with vaginal prostaglandin or expectant management. They note that induction of labour is appropriate approximately 24 hours after prelabour rupture of the membranes at term, but this appears to be more because it is custom and practice based on concerns of possible risk rather than because there is clear evidence that this improves outcomes. Infection is the main concern once the waters have broken. The amniotic fluid (waters) forms a sterile environment around the baby, and, once broken, the chance of infection increases. However, this does not mean that every baby whose waters break will get an infection, and the evidence does not show a clear difference in the outcomes of the babies born to women who decide to be induced and the outcomes of the babies born to women who decide to wait.

Dare et al (2006) reviewed 12 trials that compared planned management (induction with prostaglandin, oxytocin or, in one trial, homeopathic caullophyllum) and expectant management (waiting). They found no difference in the rate of neonatal infection or in the mode of delivery (that is, whether more women ended up having caesarean sections). More women in the waiting groups developed an infection, which is not that surprising because they had more time in which to experience this. Most of these infections were not serious. More babies born to women in the waiting groups were admitted to neonatal intensive care, but this might be because the midwives or doctors were more cautious with the babies of women who waited. Dare et al (2012: 2) concluded that *since planned and expectant management may not be very different, women need to have appropriate information to make informed choices'*.

Another study, which is older but whose results are quite helpful, was published by Savitz et al in 1997. They calculated that, for every hundred women whose waters break at term (after 37 weeks) but before labour starts and who wait,

- 86 will go into labour within the first 24 hours;

- 91 will have gone into labour by the time 48 hours have passed;

- 94 will have gone into labour by the time 96 hours have passed;

- only 6 will not be in labour within 96 hours.

Women who decide to wait and see in this situation may find they are offered certain kinds of monitoring. Although there hasn't been much research to test whether the following things actually make a difference, it may be worth being cautious in the interests of possibly reducing the risk of infection. Some things that midwives sometimes recommend are:

- Avoiding sex or putting anything in or near the vagina (including vaginal examinations). This may be something to consider when weighing up the decision to have induction or not, because induction of labour involves multiple vaginal examinations, and may entail the insertion of prostaglandin or mechanical cervical devices into the vagina. Each vaginal examination carries a risk of infection, even when sterile gloves are worn.

- Having regular showers.

- Eating a healthy diet (including lots of fruit and vegetables, ensuring adequate amounts of protein, limiting sugar and 'junk' food) and drinking plenty of water.

- Checking your temperature regularly for signs of any rise that might indicate an infection. This may be something to discuss with a midwife to get more information about.

Given the lack of evidence for routinely inducing labour at a certain stage of pregnancy, each individual woman needs to make her own decision in the light of her personal circumstances. Hospitals are likely to continue to recommend induction for the foreseeable future, despite research evidence questioning the value of this. This may be because of differences in belief systems, because it takes a long time for change to happen, because it is felt that it is better to do rather than not do, and/or because the challenge of trying to create a system that provides a service to thousands of women each year means it can be difficult to take an individualised approach to the needs of each woman.

Induction of labour in older women

In many countries, the past decade or two has seen more women having babies at a later age. For lots of reasons that we don't have room to explore here, the average age of a woman having a baby in England or Wales increased from 28.5 in 2000 to 29.5 in 2010 (Office for National Statistics 2013) and women are also giving birth to their first child later. Women who are older than average when they give birth often find that they are labelled as 'high risk' by the maternity services. They may be told they need more monitoring or intervention, and there is an increasing trend in some areas towards suggesting that their labour should be induced even earlier – sometimes as early as 40 weeks. In this section, I want to spell out what we do and do not know about this.

Firstly, I would like to quote Rosemary Mander, a midwife and researcher who wrote about the way in which there is a negative bias in this area:

'Research reports and recommendations ... tend to ignore the positive aspects of advancing maternal age. These include the likelihood that psychological and social strengths, such as increased confidence, may

more than compensate for any biological problems with which advanced age may be associated.' (Mander 2013: 49)

Rosemary was responding to a paper published by the Royal College of Obstetricians and Gynaecologists in 2013, which suggested that induction should be routinely offered to women aged 40 years or more at 39-40 weeks' gestation in the hope of reducing the rate of stillborn babies. However, this paper is not a systematic review, and it draws selectively on research studies, some of which are of poor quality.

'There are also a number of unexplained slightly paradoxical points which reduce the reader's confidence in the paper, such as the statement "that ageing impairs myometrial [uterus muscle] function" (2013). This leads the reader to question why, if this is so, are such "older mothers" being recommended to labour at all?' (Mander 2013: 48)

It is true that some studies suggest that there may be a correlation between increased maternal age and an increase in certain types of complications, but this finding is not straightforward and may even be misleading. Complications can become more likely when women experience lots of intervention and, somewhat ironically, monitoring for complications. Women who are older are often offered monitoring and intervention in abundance. Also, because practitioners are already a bit more worried about older women (often in a kindly way, for instance because they are aware that this may be the woman's last chance to have a baby or because they know it costs a lot to use assisted reproductive technologies), they may be more likely to be on the lookout for problems. This may explain why older women are more likely to have a caesarean section for 'slow labour progress' and studies by Wang et al (2011) and Carolan et al (2011) have both confirmed that there is a lower threshold for caesareans in older women. In other words, because caregivers are worried that being older is a risk factor, they tend to suggest intervention sooner than they would if the woman was younger. The intervention itself can cause more problems, such as increased bleeding, and, ultimately, a self-fulfilling prophecy is created.

The RCOG (2013) paper also states that older women have a greater chance of having a stillborn baby, but this is a very complicated claim to analyse, partly for the reasons explained in the previous paragraph. As it acknowledges, women who are older are more likely to have a pregnancy that resulted from the use of assisted reproductive technologies and they are also more likely to have a pre-existing medical or obstetric problem. All of these things can cause problems, so researchers should take them into account when they analyse the data, but in many of the studies the researchers didn't do this. The RCOG (2013) paper mentions only two studies which did control for these factors and found that the stillbirth rate is higher. The first of them is a Canadian study (Fretts et al 1995) which used data gathered from 1961 to 1993, and the second study analysed data from Scottish women (Pasupathy et al 2011). Although the second study appears to be more recent, it also looked back at older data, this time at the outcomes of women who had given birth between 1985 and 2004.

Midwifery and obstetric practice has changed in many ways since the time that the women in these studies gave birth. Also, as I said above, the reasons for the increase in average maternal age are complex, but if even some of this increase is because women are having careers first, then the older women giving birth today may be very different from the older women who were giving birth in the 1980s. Some of them might, for instance, have more money, which might in turn lead to them being better nourished and in better health. Or it might not! They might eat more organic food than their 1980s counterparts but be more stressed and have less time to relax! Women need to think about their own individual circumstances in relation to this point, and whether the results of studies which were carried out on a possibly very different population of women who gave birth up to fifty years ago will be relevant to them.

One further point to consider is that Pasupathy et al (2011) argued that the increase in stillbirths in women over 40 was the result of anoxia (which means a lack of oxygen for the baby). Yet it again seems illogical to suggest that the answer to this is induction of labour, because one of the risks of synthetic oxytocin is that it can cause a lack of oxygen for the baby. This point is similar to the one that Rosemary Mander made about the claim that the uterine muscle is inefficient; if these things are really of concern, then induction of labour isn't the most logical solution to either. (This point has been discussed further at sarawickham.com/2013/11/24/birthillogics-1-induction-for-advanced-maternal-age/ if you are interested.)

I understand that it is not a very helpful conclusion, but I do not believe that we have good enough data in this area to make clear-cut recommendations based on research. It then comes down to what people believe, and we already know that the default position of the maternity services is that it is generally better to intervene than not, just in case. I do not believe the data show that advancing maternal age is the clear-cut problem that some people claim, but I also want to be clear that I am not saying that giving birth at an older age is without risk. It is more complex than that, and there are too many things that we do not know. As Rosemary Mander argued, being older also comes with benefits, which are largely ignored in the literature. In addition, even if being older does carry more risk, we do not have good evidence to show that induction of labour will reduce those risks. I am aware that further research is planned, although, at the time of publishing, I am concerned that it is going to be used to suggest that women at the younger age of 35 should be induced earlier.

Non-medical induction of labour

There are a number of time-honoured ways in which women attempt to encourage their labours to start, including eating certain foods (for example hot curry, dates, fresh pineapple), riding down bumpy roads in the car or bouncing on a birth ball, having a glass of wine or taking a brisk walk. Other examples – including making love, hugging, touch and massage – are thought to help stimulate the release of natural prostaglandins and oxytocin, which is released when we are involved in such activities. Oxytocin release is inhibited by the hormone adrenalin, which is released when we feel unsafe, are stressed or are engaging in hard exercise. Whether or not these things work to stimulate labour is perhaps secondary to the fact that they are things that women might do anyway, and they are unlikely to do any harm.

Some women also know (or are told by their midwives) that there are non-medical ways of inducing labour which might be more effective, such as acupuncture, homeopathy, herbs and reflexology. These methods might be seen as an alternative to spending the early part of labour in a hospital and can be an attractive alternative to women who want their labour to start, but without the drugs, monitoring or interference which are often involved in the process of medical induction.

Cochrane reviewers have attempted to evaluate some of these methods, but most have not been tested for effectiveness and safety in research trials, perhaps primarily because they are not valued by the sort of bodies that allocate money for medical research and there is little money to be made from them because they can't be patented. Generally the reviewers conclude that they are either not effective or that there is not enough evidence to make this decision. It is worth noting that many alternative therapies do not come out well when evaluated by the research tools of western medicine anyway, because alternative therapies are often personalised, whereas medical research trials require standardised diagnoses and treatments. Also, as has been discussed already in this book, some aspects of the medical methods of induction have not always been tested as rigorously as you might suppose either.

The decision to try a method of non-medical induction of labour is often made in response to the pressure put on women to accept medical inductions they would rather avoid. Any method to try to induce should be carefully considered because of the effect on the baby and because the baby may not be ready to be born (see page 68 for more on dating pregnancy). I have written a couple of articles about this for midwives (Wickham 2012a, 2012b) and in them I have challenged the term 'natural induction' because I think it is an oxymoron.

I absolutely understand why some women try non-medical methods of induction, however, and I know this can be a positive choice for some women. These methods can enable women to have the home birth they planned, or to retain some control over the early part of their labour before they go to hospital once strong contractions are established. They can make the difference between feeling very pressured because a hospital-imposed deadline is looming, and feeling that you are taking some control back. The choice of non-medical induction is a very personal one and you might like to explore some of the different methods and think just as carefully about the issues surrounding this option as you would about medical induction. But please don't try it just because you feel you have no choice or because you feel that you have to consent to unwanted medical induction otherwise. You can say no, or you can say you want to wait and see, and AIMS is here to support you if this is what you want to do and you need help.

A Final Word

This book has explored some of the complex issues surrounding what has become a very common intervention at the end of pregnancy. Midwives and doctors do not understand the mechanism by which labour starts, although it is known that it is the baby itself who triggers labour. Many women feel that they would rather trust their baby to arrive when it is ready rather than rushing it into the world with synthetic drugs based on estimates that may not be accurate. Others feel that induction of labour is a positive choice that is right for them.

There are pros and cons to be considered for most of the decisions you will make about what's best for your baby during the childbearing year and for many years to come, and whether or not to have an induction is no exception. The bottom line piece of advice should be to get as much relevant information as possible and then make a decision that feels right for you, rather than going along with what anybody else thinks. The references in the following section provide ideas of where to go if you would like to follow up some of the things discussed here in more depth.

If you do choose induction, then I hope this book has helped you to understand a bit more about what will happen, and perhaps given you a sense of having more control. If you decide not to have induction, or to delay the decision, then I hope this book has helped you to gain more information to support that decision. If you feel you are being pushed into a decision, then I really hope you can find tools in here that will help you to work out what is right for **you**.

Finally, if you are reading this because you have been given a date for induction of labour at an antenatal appointment or in a way that makes you feel that you can't challenge it and you later realise that you are not happy with this, I hope you know now that you are entitled to change your mind if you want to. Whatever your situation, the maternity services are there to meet your needs, not the other way around! You (or your partner or a friend) can call your midwife, doctor, clinic or hospital and change any decision. You could consider getting a second opinion, perhaps by calling the hospital and asking to speak to a Supervisor of Midwives.

You can always call or email AIMS for advice or support, whatever decision you have made. Please consider becoming a member of AIMS, as this will enable you to access information and updates through AIMS Journal and the members forum, and your membership will help us continue to produce information to help other women who are making decisions now and in the future.

Thank you.

References

This reference list contains the articles, papers and studies that are cited and referred to in this book. Where a resource such as a Cochrane review has been updated, I have usually only included the most recent version unless I specifically referred to different versions in the text of the book. The Cochrane Library contains comprehensive details of the publication history of all reviews.

Anderson T (2000). How to calculate an EDD. The Practising Midwife 3(3): 12-13.

Bakker JJH, van der Goes BY, Pel M, Mol BWJ, van der Post JAM (2013). Morning versus evening induction of labour for improving outcomes. Cochrane Database of Systematic Reviews 2013, Issue 2: CD007707. doi: 10/1002/14651858.CD007707.pub2.

Baud D, Rouiller S, Hohlfeld P, Tolsa J-F, Vial Y (2013). Adverse obstetrical and neonatal outcomes in elective and medically indicated inductions of labor at term. The Journal of Maternal-Fetal and Neonatal Medicine 26(16): 1595-1601. doi: 10.3109/14767058.2013.795533.

Beech B (2004). Who says ultrasound is safe? AIMS Journal 16(4): 10-11.

Berkowitz RL (2011). Of parachutes and patient care: a call to action. American Journal of Obstetrics and Gynecology 205(1): 7-9. doi: 10.1016/j.ajog.2010.12.020.

Boulvain M, Stan CM, Irion O (2005). Membrane sweeping for induction of labour. Cochrane Database of Systematic Reviews 2005, Issue 1. Art. No.: CD000451. doi: 10.1002/14651858.CD000451.pub2.

Buchanan SL, Crowther CA, Levett KM, Middleton P, Morris J (2010). Planned early birth versus expectant management for women with prelabour rupture of membranes prior to 37 weeks' gestation for improving pregnancy outcome. Cochrane Database of Systematic Reviews 2010, Issue 3, Art. No.: CD004735. doi: 10.1002/14651858.CD004735.pub3.

Buckley S (2009). Gentle Birth, Gentle Mothering: A Doctor's Guide to Natural Childbirth and Gentle Early Parenting Choices. Celestial Arts. A related article is freely available at www.sarahbuckley.com/pain-in-labour-your-hormones-are-your-helpers/ and several of Sarah's articles can be found at www.sarahbuckley.com.

Carolan M, Davey M-A, Biro MA, Kealy M (2011). Older maternal age and intervention in labor: a population-based study comparing older and younger first-time mothers in Victoria, Australia. Birth 38(1): 24-29.

Cotzias CS, Paterson-Brown S, Fisk NM (1999). Prospective risk of unexplained stillbirth in singleton pregnancies at term: population based analysis. BMJ 319(7205): 287-288. doi: 10.1136/bmj.319.7205.287.

Dare MR, Middleton P, Crowther CA, Flenady V, Varatharaju B (2006). Planned early birth versus expectant management (waiting) for prelabour rupture of membranes at term (37 weeks or more).

Cochrane Database of Systematic Reviews 2006, Issue 1. Art. No.: CD005302. doi: 10.1002/14651858.CD005302.pub2.

Edwards N (2008). Women's Emotion Work in the Context of Current Maternity Services. In: Hunter B and Deery R. Emotions in Midwifery and Reproduction. Palgrave, London.

Edwards NP, Wickham S (2011). Birthing Your Placenta: The Third Stage. AIMS

Fretts RC, Schmittdiel J, McLean FH, Usher RH, Goldman MB (1995). Increased maternal age and the risk of fetal death. New England Journal of Medicine 333: 953–957. doi: 10.1056/NEJM199510123331501.

Glantz JC (2012). Obstetric variation, intervention, and outcomes: doing more but accomplishing less. Birth 39(4): 286-290. doi: 10.1111/12002.

Gülmezoglu AM, Crowther CA, Middleton P, Heatley E (2012). Induction of labour for improving birth outcomes for women at or beyond term. Cochrane Database of Systematic Reviews 2012, Issue 6. Art. No.: CD004945. doi: 10.1002/14651858.CD004945.pub3.

Hannah ME, Hannah WJ, Hellman J, Hewson S, Milner R, Willan A (1992). The Canadian Multicenter Post-term Pregnancy Trial Group: Induction of labour as compared with serial antenatal monitoring in post-term pregnancy. New England Journal of Medicine, 326 (24): 1587-1592. doi: 10.1056/NEJM199206113262402

Heimstad R, Romundstad PR, Salvesen KA (2008). Induction of labour for post-term pregnancy and risk estimates for intrauterine and perinatal death. Acta Obstetricia et Gynecologica Scandinavica 87: 247-249. doi: 10.1080/00016340701743165.

Henry A, Madan A, Reid R, Tracy SK, Austin K, Welsh A, Challis D (2013). Outpatient Foley catheter versus inpatient prostaglandin E2 gel for induction of labour: a randomised trial. BMC Pregnancy and Childbirth 13: 25 doi:10.1186/1471-2393-13-25.

Hilder L, Costeloe K, Thilaganathan B (1998). Prolonged pregnancy: evaluating gestation-specific risks of fetal and infant mortality. BJOG: An International Journal of Obstetrics & Gynaecology 105: 169–173. doi: 10.1111/j.1471-0528.1998.tb10047.x.

Hussain AA, Yakoob MY, Imdad A, Bhutta ZA (2011). Elective induction for pregnancies at or beyond 41 weeks of gestation and its impact on stillbirths: a systematic review with meta-analysis. BMC Public Health. 11 (Suppl 3): S5. doi:10.1186/1471-2458-11-S3-S5.

Jozwiak M, Rengerink KO, Benthem M, et al. (2011). Foley catheter versus vaginal prostaglandin E2 gel for induction of labour at term (PROBAAT trial): an open-label, randomised controlled trial. The Lancet Volume 378, Issue 9809: 2095–103. doi: 10.1016/S0140-6736(11)61484-0.

Jozwiak M, Bloemenkamp KWM, Kelly AJ, Mol BWJ, Irion O, Boulvain M (2012). Mechanical methods for induction of labour. Cochrane Database of Systematic Reviews 2012, Issue 3. Art. No.: CD001233. doi: 10.1002/14651858.CD001233.pub2.

Jukic AM, Baird DD, Weinberg CR, McConnaughey DR, Wilcox AJ (2013). Length of human pregnancy and contributors to its natural variation. Human Reproduction 28(10): 2848-55. doi: 10.1093/humrep/det297.

Keirse MJNC, (2010). Elective induction, selective deduction, and cesarean section. Birth 37(3): 252-256.   doi: 10.1111/j.1523-536X.2010.00413.x.

Khambalia AZ, Roberts CL, Nguyen M, Algert S, Nicholl MC, Morris J (2013). Predicting date of birth and examining the best time to date a pregnancy. International Journal of Gynecology & Obstetrics 123(2): 105-109, doi:10.1016/j.ijgo.2013.05.007.

Korte D and Scaer R (1984). A Good Birth, A Safe Birth. Bantam, New York.

ISD Scotland (2013). Birth statistics. www.isdscotland.org/Health-Topics/Maternity-and-Births/Publications/

Lie RT, Wilcox AJ, Skjaerven R (2006). Maternal and paternal influences on length of pregnancy. Obstetrics and Gynecology 107(4): 880-885. doi: 10.1097/01.AOG.0000206797.52832.36.

Liu S, Joseph KS, Hutcheon JA, Bartholomew S, León JA, Walker M, et al (2013). Gestational age–specific severe maternal morbidity associated with labor induction. American Journal of Obstetrics and Gynecology 2013: 209:209.e1-8. doi:10.1016/j.ajog.2013.05.033

Lothian JA, (2006). Saying "no" to induction. Journal of Perinatal Education 15(2):   43-45.   Freely   available   online   at www.ncbi.nlm.nih.gov/pmc/articles/PMC1595289/.
doi:10.1624/105812406X107816

Mander R (2013). Induction of labour for advancing maternal age. Essentially MIDIRS 4(8): 46-49.

Mandruzzato G, Alfirevic Z, Chervenak F, Gruenebaum A, Heimstad R, Heinonen S, et al (2010). Guidelines for the management of postterm pregnancy. Journal of Perinatal Medicine 38(2): 111-9. doi: 10.1515/JPM.2010.057.

Menticoglou SM, Hall PF (2002). Routine induction of labour at 41 weeks gestation: nonsensus consensus. BJOG: An International Journal of Obstetrics and Gynaecology 109(5): 485-491. doi: 10.1111/j.1471-0528.2002.01004.x.

Mittendorf R, Williams MA, Berkey CSS, Cotter PF (1990). The length of uncomplicated human gestation. Obstetrics and Gynecology 75(6): 929-932.

Mittendorf R, Williams MA, Berkey CS, Lieberman E, Monson RR (1993). Predictors of human gestational length. American Journal of Obstetrics and Gynecology 168(2): 480-484. doi: 10.1016/0002-9378(93)90476-Y.

Moore WMO, Mittendorf R, Williams MA, Stronge JM, Rasmussen MJ (1991) Naegele's Rule (correspondence) The Lancet, 337(8746): 910. doi:10.1016/0140-6736(91)90236-I.

Murphy-Lawless, Jo (1998). Reading Birth and Death: A History of Obstetric Thinking. Cork University Press, Cork.

NHS Maternity Statistics, England: 2012-13 can be found on the Health and Social Care Information Centre website at www.hscic.gov.uk/catalogue/PUB12744/nhs-mate-eng-2012-13-summ-repo-rep.pdf

NICE (2008). Induction of Labour. RCOG, London. www.nice.org.uk/nicemedia/live/12012/41255/41255.pdf

NICE (2013a). Induction of Labour Pathway pathways.nice.org.uk/pathways/induction-of-labour#content=view-node%3Anodes-information-and-decision-making.

NICE (2013b). Induction of Labour Evidence Update July 2013. A summary of selected new evidence relevant to NICE clinical guideline 70 'Induction of labour' (2008). Evidence Update 44.

Odent M (2009). Margaret Thatcher and oxytocin. Primal Health Research 11(4): 1-8.

Odent M (2010a). Unasked questions about synthetic oxytocin. Primal Health Research 18(1): 1-7.

Odent M (2010b). If I were the baby - questioning the widespread use of synthetic oxytocin. Midwifery Today (94): 22-23.

Office for National Statistics (2013). Characteristics of mother, England and Wales - 2011. Accessible from www.statistics.gov.uk/hub/population/births-and-fertility/live-births-and-stillbirths.

Olesen AW, Westergaard JG, Olsen J (2003). Perinatal and maternal complications related to postterm delivery: a national register-based study, 1978-1993. American Journal of Obstetrics and Gynecology. 189(1): 222-227. doi: 10.1067/mob.2003.446.

Oteri O and Tasker M (1997). Get set and go: conventional action. New Generation, December: 10-11.

Pasupathy D, Wood AM, Pell JP, Fleming M, Smith GCS (2011). Advanced maternal age and the risk of perinatal death due to intrapartum anoxia at term. Journal of Epidemiology and Community Health 65(3): 241–245. doi:10.1136/jech.2009.097170

Porter M, Macintyre S (1984). What is, must be best: a research note on conservative or deferential responses to antenatal care provision. Social Science and Medicine. 19(11): 1197-200. doi: 10.1016/0277-9536(84)90370-8.

Robinson J (2000). Ultrasound - more powerful, more dangerous, more unethical. AIMS Journal 11(4): 13-15.

Rosser J (2000). Calculating the EDD: which is more accurate, scan or LMP? The Practising Midwife, 3(3): 28-29.

RCOG (2001). Induction of Labour. Evidence-Based Clinical Guideline 9. RCOG Press, London.

RCOG (2013). Induction of Labour at Term in Older Mothers. Scientific Impact Paper. 34. RCOG, London.

Saunders N, Paterson C (1991). Can we abandon Naegele's rule? The Lancet, 337(8741): 600-601. doi: 10.1016.0140-6736(91)91653-C.

Savitz DA, Ananth CV, Luther ER, Thorp JM (1997). Influence of gestational age on the time from spontaneous rupture of the chorioamniotic membranes to the onset of labour. American Journal of Perinatology. 14(3): 129-133. doi: 10/1055/s-2007s994112.

Sentilhes L, Bouet PE, Mezzadri M, Combaud V, Madzou S, Biquard F et al (2011). Assessment of the benefit-harm balance depending on gestational age to induce delivery for post-term pregnancies. Journal de Gynecologie Obstetrique et Biologie de la Reproduction (Paris). 40(8): 747-66. doi: 10/1016/j.jgyn.2011.09.019. [Article in French]

Simpson KR, Thorman KE, (2005). Obstetric "conveniences": elective induction of labor, cesarean birth on demand, and other potentially unnecessary interventions. Journal of Perinatal and Neonatal Nursing 19(2): 134-144.

Uvnäs-Moberg K (2011). The Oxytocin Factor – Tapping the Hormone of Calm, Love and Healing. Pinter and Martin, London.

van der Ham DP, Vijgen SMC, Nijhuis JG, van Beek JJ, Opmeer BC, Mulder ALM, et al. (2012a). Induction of labor versus expectant management in women with preterm prelabor rupture of membranes between 34 and 37 weeks: a randomized controlled trial. PLOS Medicine 9: e1001208 doi: 10.1371/journal.pmed.1001208

van der Ham DP, van der Heyden JL, Opmeer BC, Mulder ALM, Moonen MJ, van Beek JJ, et al. (2012b). Management of late-preterm premature rupture of membranes: the PPROMEXIL-2 trial. American Journal of Obstetrics and Gynecology 207(4): 276.e1-276.e10. doi: 10.1016/j.ajog.2012.07.024

van der Kooy B (1994). Calculating expected date of delivery – its accuracy and relevance. Midwifery Matters 60: 4-7,24.

van Teijlingen, ER, Hundley V, Rennie A-M, Graham W, Fitzmaurice A (2003). Maternity satisfaction studies and their limitations: "What Is, Must Still Be Best". Birth 30: 75-82. doi: 10.1046/j.1523-536X.2003.00224.x.

Verhoeven CJM, Opmeer BC, Oei SG, Latour V, van der Post JA, Mol BW (2013). Transvaginal sonographic assessment of cervical length and wedging for predicting outcome of labor induction at term: a systematic review and meta-analysis. Ultrasound in Obstetrics and Gynecology 42(5): 500-508. doi: 10.1002/uog.12467

Wang Y, Tanbo T, Abyholm T, Henriksen T (2011). The impact of advanced maternal age and parity on obstetric and perinatal outcomes in singleton gestations. Archives of Gynecology and Obstetrics 284(1): 31–37. doi: 10.1007/s00404-010-1587-x.

Wennerholm U-B, Hagberg H, Brorsson B, Bergh C (2009). Induction of labor versus expectant management for postdate pregnancy: is there sufficient evidence for a change in clinical practice? Acta Scandinavica Obstetricia et Gynecologica 88(1): 6–17. doi: 10.1080/00016340802555948.

Whitworth M, Bricker L, Neilson JP, Dowswell T (2010). Ultrasound for fetal assessment in early pregnancy. Cochrane Database of Systematic Reviews 14(4): CD007058. doi: 10.1002/14651858.CD007058.pub2.

Wickham S (2007). Jenna's care story: post-term pregnancy. In: L Page and R McCandlish. The New Midwifery: Science and Sensitivity in Practice. Elsevier, Oxford.

Wickham S (2009). Post-term pregnancy: the problem of the boundaries. MIDIRS Midwifery Digest 19(4): 463-469. sarawickham.files.wordpress.com/2011/10/a1e-post-term-pregnancy-the-problem-of-the-boundaries.pdf.

Wickham S (2010). Journeying with women: holistic midwives and relationship. Birthspirit Midwifery Journal 6, 15-21.

Wickham S (2011). Stretching the fabric: from technocratic normal limits to holistic midwives' negotiations of normalcy. Essentially MIDIRS 2(11):17-23. sarawickham.files.wordpress.com/2013/04/em-stretching-the-fabric.pdf

Wickham S (2012a). When is induction not induction? Essentially MIDIRS 3(9): 50-51.

Wickham S (2012b). The continuum of induction. Essentially MIDIRS 3(10): 50-51

World Health Organisation, Deptartment of Reproductive Health and Research (WHO) (2011). WHO Recommendations for Induction of labour. www.who.int/reproductivehealth/publications/maternal_perinatal_health/9789241501156/en/.

Yamada T, Cho K, Yamada T, Morikawa M, Minakami H (2013). Labor induction by transcervical balloon catheter and cerebral palsy associated with umbilical cord prolapse. The Journal of Obstetrics and Gynaecology Research 39(6): 1159-1164. doi: 10.1111/jog.12036. Epub 2013 Apr 3.

Yeh P, Emary K, Impey L (2012). The relationship between umbilical cord arterial pH and serious adverse neonatal outcome: analysis of 51,519 consecutive validated samples. BJOG: An International Journal of Obstetrics & Gynaecology 119(7): 824-831. doi: 10.1111/j.1471-0528.2012.03335.x.

Contents

www.aims.org.uk
Twitter @AIMS_online
Facebook www.facebook.com/AIMSUK

Helpline 0300 365 0663
helpline@aims.org.uk